Your Career
in Nursing

Other Kaplan Books for Nurses

NCLEX-PN®: Strategies for the Practical Nursing Licensing Exam

NCLEX-RN®: Strategies for the Registered Nursing Licensing Exam

NCLEX-RN® Exam: Medication in a Box

Your Career in Nursing

Fourth Edition

Annette Vallano, M.S., R.N., A.P.R.N., B.C.

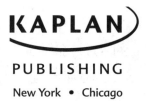

KAPLAN PUBLISHING

New York • Chicago

Published by Kaplan Publishing, a division of Kaplan, Inc.
888 Seventh Ave.
New York, NY 10106

Kaplan® is a registered trademark of Kaplan, Inc.

NCLEX-RN® is a registered trademark of the National Council of State Boards of Nursing, which neither sponsors nor endorses this product.

Bennet Swingle, Anne. "Still Not Much of a Guy Thing." *Hopkins Medicine* (a publication of the Johns Hopkins Medical Institute). By permission of the author.

Cataldo, Jackie. "Smoke and Debris" Reprinted with permission from the *Journal of the New York State Nurses Association,* Spring/Summer 2002, Volume 33, Number 1.

Shihab Nye, Naomi. "The Art of Disappearing." By permission of the author.

Williams, Michael. "President's Notes: A Journey of Rediscovery: So How Does it Feel to You?" *AACN News,* August 2001. By permission of the author.

Wilson, Bruce, R.N., Ph. D. "Men in American Nursing History," *www.geocities.com/~brucewilson*. By permission of the author.

"Nursing. It's real. It's life." Courtesy of Nurses for a Healthier Tomorrow.

"Be a nurse." Courtesy of Johnson & Johnson, Inc., The Campaign for Nursing's Future.

Contributing Editors: Judith A. Burckhardt, Ph.D., R.N.
Editorial Director: Jennifer Farthing
Project Editor: Anne Kemper
Production Editor: Michael Hankes
Production Artist: Virginia Byrne
Cover Designer: Carly Schnur

Manufactured in the United States of America.
Published simultaneously in Canada.

10 9 8 7 6 5 4 3 2 1

December 2006

ISBN-13: 978-1-4195-5062-1
ISBN-10:   1-4195-5062-4

Kaplan Publishing books are available at special quantity discounts to use for sales promotions, employee premiums, or educational purposes. Please call our Special Sales Department to order or for more information at 800-621-9621, ext. 4444, e-mail kaplanpubsales@kaplan.com, or write to Kaplan Publishing, 30 South Wacker Drive, Suite 2500, Chicago, IL 60606-7481.

TABLE OF CONTENTS

ABOUT THE AUTHOR

Annette T. Vallano, M.S., R.N., A.P.R.N., B.C., is a clinical nurse specialist in psychiatric mental-health nursing and is in private practice in New York City. Her longstanding interest in and commitment to the professional and personal well-being of nurses has shaped and influenced the direction of her career for more than 25 years, and continues to provide the foundation of her psychotherapy and career-coaching practice, her organizational consulting, and the undergraduate nursing course in self-care she teaches at Mercy College. In addition, Annette is studying to become a psychoanalyst at the Institute for Contemporary Psychotherapy in New York.

Annette has transformed her nursing career many times. A diploma graduate of St. John's Episcopal Hospital in Brooklyn, New York, she went on to receive her B.S.N. and M.S. from Adelphi University. She has been a direct care nurse, a nurse manager, a nurse educator, and a nurse psychotherapist working in pediatrics, women's health, and psychiatric mental-health nursing in a variety of organizations, including the U.S. Army Nurse Corps. Her extensive nursing experience gives her first hand knowledge of the complexities, challenges, and rewards of nursing practice.

CONTRIBUTORS

Karen A. Ballard, M.A., R.N., is a nurse consultant in private practice specializing in professional practice issues and health policy. She is the co-chair of the Nurses Workgroup for Health Care Without Harm, an international coalition of 433 organizations in 52 countries working to make the healthcare industry environmentally responsible. Previously, for 20 years, Ms. Ballard held various staff positions with the New York State Nurses Association including Director of Special Projects and Director of the Practice and Governmental Affairs Program where she interpreted nursing practice issues, served as a lobbyist, and addressed such issues as bioterrorism, HIV/AIDS, reimbursement, nursing acuity, and the nursing shortage. Ms. Ballard has her bachelor's degree in nursing from Niagara University and her master's degree in child and adolescent psychiatric-mental health nursing from New York University. Her recent publications include a textbook, *Psychiatric Nursing—An Integration of Theory and Practice*, and articles on "Patient Safety: A Shared Responsibility" in *Online Journal of Issues in Nursing* and "Measuring Variations in Nursing Care Across DRGs" in *Nursing Management*. She authored Chapter 2 of this book, "The World of Nursing Practice."

Contributors (Cont.)

Alayne Fitzpatrick, A.P.R.N., B.C., Ed.D., is the associate director of the nursing programs at Mercy College where she has taught for over 20 years in the classroom and online. As a coordinator of online education for the undergraduate nursing program she works with faculty, administration, and students; as a consultant she works with healthcare providers and educators on technology usage. She received her doctorate from Columbia University. She has published extensively, and contributed to Chapter 4 of this book, "The Nurse and Technology."

Mary McGuinness, R.N., Ph.D., is director of the Nursing Programs at Mercy College, New York. Dr. McGuinness has been a nursing educator for over 20 years and earned her Ph.D. in Nursing from New York University. Dr. McGuinness has been an advocate and mentor for students in baccalaureate, R.N. to B.S.N., and master's programs for over 30 years. A consultant in curriculum development, she has developed and implemented several innovative nursing programs. She contributed to Chapter 3 of this book, "The State of Nursing Education."

AUTHOR'S PREFACE

There has never been a better time to be a nurse or to consider nursing as a career. The nursing shortage, the influence of managed care and computer technology are reshaping the healthcare landscape and filling its many workplaces with opportunities and challenges for all those willing to embrace change and plant both feet firmly in a 21st-century world.

In writing this book, I hoped you would find the information and support you would need to make intelligent choices about your career and to feel invigorated about what you can contribute. Opportunities abound, and each segment of the nursing profession has something important to contribute:

> **The newly graduated nurse** contributes a contagious infusion of new energy and bright idealism, and a desire to learn that enlivens all those with whom they come in contact.
>
> **The second-career nurse** brings invaluable maturity and enthusiasm in the achievement of a long-sought goal, along with a fresh perspective drawn on valuable prior work experience.
>
> **Men who become nurses** bring an important dynamic to the profession, balancing its traditional gender roles and creating a true 21st-century nursing practice.
>
> **The older nurse,** whether currently working or retired, can contribute his or her years of wisdom, nursing skills, and competencies, acting as a preceptor, mentor, or coach.
>
> **Every nurse,** across all generations, genders, and cultures has a sphere of influence in which to make a unique contribution. It may be your nursing skills and competencies, your proficiency with technology, your ability to teach, or any of the many other talents and abilities I know you have.

The changes facing us in the 21st century require information, insight, and resilience. I've worked side by side with you for many years, in many capacities. I know the *obstacles* you face, and I know your ability to transform these obstacles into challenges and to conquer them.

I honor and support the depth of your caring and the strength of your power. I hope you will use the winds of change to set sail in the direction of making your voice heard and your actions matter.

Dedication

To the enduring and supportive memory of Evelyn Zalewski, M.A., R.N., nurse, teacher, mentor, healer, with eternal gratitude and affection, and to Hilda and Jim, across the bridges of time, with renewed love and ongoing appreciation.

PART ONE

The Healthcare Landscape of the 21st Century

CHAPTER 1

The 21st-Century Nurse

As the 21st century unfolds, we live amid the inheritance of the previous century's jolting changes, the horror of the September 11, 2001 attack on America, the war in Iraq that followed, the December 2004 tsunami disaster in South Asia, and the devastation of the U.S. Gulf Coast by Hurricane Katrina in 2005. The 1990s saw the birth and rapid growth of the age of information, in which technology exploded into our lives, and computers transformed how we used and accessed information, and the connections we made to one another as a result. The proliferation of fax machines, cell phones, and email created new communication possibilities that blurred the boundaries between work time and personal time, a phenomenon as exciting as it was overwhelming. The turbulent '90s created a stressful state of paradox that became the psychological hallmark of that time, and ours as well.

> "Our deepest fear is not that we are inadequate. Our deepest fear is that we are powerful beyond measure. It is our light, not our darkness, that most frightens us. We ask ourselves, who am I to be brilliant, gorgeous, talented, and fabulous? Actually, who are you not to be? You are a child of God. Your playing small doesn't serve the world. . . . As we are liberated from our own fear, our presence automatically liberates others."
>
> —*Nelson Mandela, from his 1994 inaugural speech*

THE HEALTHCARE REVOLUTION

The 1990s were also the beginning of the healthcare revolution, in which historical as well as social, political, and economic factors led to the onset of managed care with its fiscal restraint. Managed care in turn led to organizational reengineering and the era of downsizing, in which job security was threatened for millions, including nurses, for the first time in the history of that profession. Interestingly, despite the artificial surplus of nurses created by the economic necessity of downsizing, there was *still* a nursing shortage that was growing more severe as the 1990s marched on and as the healthcare needs of many segments of the population, including aging baby boomers, increased. This nursing shortage is predicted to deepen as the 21st century marches on. You can count on it to impact your work as a nurse, as well as to influence the quality of healthcare people receive. Information about the nursing shortage is woven throughout this book, particularly in Chapter 2, "The World of Nursing Practice," and Chapter 11, "The Market Research Department of *You, Inc.*"

ON THE EDGE OF TRANSFORMATION

The world of work, including the work of nurses, has been and will continue to be transformed by these events and by the exciting new frontiers of health and medicine just now becoming known at the beginning of this century. The description below appeared in *Newsweek* (6/24/02) as an introduction to its special report on health and medicine titled "Medicine and Technology: What the Future Means for You—The Next Frontiers." As you read it, imagine how these breakthroughs will influence *your* future as a nurse. See a glimpse into the not too distant future of healthcare, and of what might be required of professionals in it.

"How does the brain work, and why does it fail? An old medical mystery is yielding to new technologies. Scientists can now inspect, repair, and sometimes even replace dysfunctional parts of the nervous system. Advances in biotechnology and computerized brain scans mean that doctors can detect Alzheimer's earlier, and may lead to treatments that slow the course of this tragic disease. Researchers are working on 'neural prostheses,' which, like the prosthetic limbs that help amputees, may allow patients with impaired organs to regain the ability to speak, hear, and see. And an astonishing technique called 'deep-brain stimulation' is showing great promise in treating Parkinson's disease and other neurological disorders; it may also have potential in countering obsessive-compulsive disorder."

"This array of new technologies has changed what doctors need to know, and how they are learning it. The days of studying anatomy by dissecting a cadaver may soon be over. Computerized models simulate all kinds of diseases, injuries, and even responses to drugs or surgery. Med school students are wired as well, downloading critical information from their ubiquitous PDAs. In the revolutionary field of bionanotechnology, doctors foresee the day when they'll be fighting cancer, AIDS, and diabetes by delivering drugs to the specific cells that need them. In the war against disease, technology is an increasingly powerful weapon. The objective: better health, longer lives."[1]

As these new technologies "change what doctors need to know," you can count on a parallel change in what nurses need to know. If "med school students are wired," so will be the nursing school students. Chapter 4, "The Nurse and Technology," will discuss the important influence of and relationship with technology that every 21st-century nurse will experience.

REEVALUATING VALUES

We are indeed living in a world hard to imagine only a decade ago. Horrific tragedies including the September 11, 2001 attack, the war in Iraq, the tsunami in South Asia, and Hurricane Katrina have changed our world. As a result, we find ourselves grappling with questions of liberty, freedom, and how civilized people are supposed to respond and behave. On a personal level we are rethinking our values, our priorities, the meaning we want our lives to have, and the way in which we want to spend our time. We are more keenly aware of the unpredictability of life, and are taking a second look at the quality of our careers, our work lives, and our relationships. Rhema Ellis, reporting for NBC News (*The News with Brian Williams*, 6/7/02), summarized the essence of this reevaluation after she interviewed a cross-section of the nation's 2002 graduating classes and reported the following:

> "Graduates are asking themselves, 'How can I help?' rather than 'What do I want?' They are less preoccupied with indulgence and more focused on reflection; they are feeling a greater responsibility to making a contribution to the world. Many are more interested in employment in the nonprofit world than in corporate America. There is a shift in predominant life values as reflected in a concern with who one has in one's life rather than what one has. Many are expressing a desire to make a difference, to do more than just have a job. Whether or not the graduate has changed their career path as a result of 9/11, most have committed themselves to be more effective in their daily life."[2]

Many, if not all the desires and concerns expressed by these graduates, including the life and work values they want, are and always have been embodied in the profession of nursing. The desire "to make a difference, to do more than just have a job" is what often brings people into nursing to begin with. This life-affirming value, which is characteristic of being a nurse, is captured in the phrase, *"Nursing. It's real. It's life!"* During the spring of 2002, this phrase was flashed across the movie screens of selected cities as part of a print and television campaign developed by Nurses for a Healthier Tomorrow, a coalition of nearly 40 national nursing and healthcare organizations, including the National Student Nurses' Association and the Honor Society of Nursing, Sigma Theta Tau. The campaign is

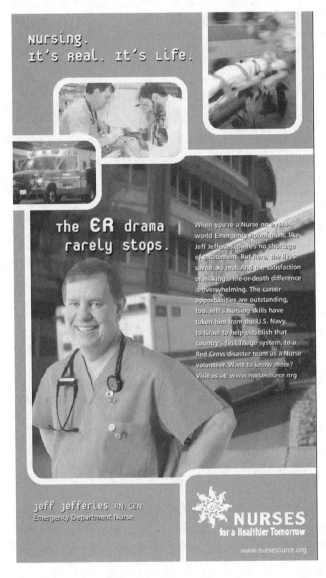

designed to encourage young people to enter the field of nursing. (See *nursesource.org* for information about the campaign and about nursing as well).

Making a contribution to the world, making a difference in the lives of others, doing work that is more than just a job . . . this is what nurses do every day. They are witness to and participants in the pain and sorrow, joy and exhilaration, and life and death that are part of the human condition.

THE ESSENCE OF NURSING

To touch others and to be touched in return: this is the essence of nursing. Nurses express and enact this life-affirming philosophy in diverse ways. For example, U.S. Army Captain Brian Gegel, a nurse anesthetist, felt his time in Iraq gave him a gift. He said, "You appreciate the freedoms our country offers, which are often taken for granted. You realize many day-to-day problems are not so important. I try to be a better person." (Reprinted with permission from *Report*, The Official Newsletter of NYSNA, February 2005, Vol. 35, No. 2.)

Many nurses who served with relief organizations following the South Asian tsunami described their experiences as a source of personal growth. You can read about their experiences at *nurseweek.com*.

Nurses were front and center during the catastrophe that befell the nation's Gulf Coast during Hurricane Katrina and in its aftermath. They were seen refusing to abandon patients who could not be evacuated, caring for patients on life support who were being airlifted to safety, and obtaining leave from their jobs across the country to volunteer their services. For moving and inspiring personal accounts of the experiences of nurses in the Gulf Coast region during and following Hurricane Katrina, log on to *nursingspectrum.com/katrina*.

Jackie Cataldo, B.S.N., R.N., is a nursing representative and organizer for the New York State Nurses Association, as well as an American Red Cross volunteer who serves on the Brooklyn Disaster Assistance Team. She wrote the poem on the next page, which is among five of her reflections about September 11, 2001, written as poems.

The other poems, along with additional stories about the role of nurses on that day and thereafter, as well as scholarly articles written by nurses about responses to crises and disasters can be found in the *Journal of the New York State Nurses Association*, Spring/Summer 2002 (*nysna.org*).

While the smoke and debris of Jackie Cataldo's poem is about September 11th, it is also symbolically representative of the experiences that nurses have with people whose lives are being dismantled by illness and injury.

Smoke and Debris

Smoke and debris
Swirling mist in the artificial light.
Eeriness prevails the night.

Hell living through this tragedy.
Living?
Bodies mingled with concrete and steel.
Shattered glass and shreds of clothing.
Our mothers, fathers, sisters, brothers
and friends gone.
Breath crushed, seared from their lungs,
Hearts and children left alone. Pain.
Insurmountable pain for the buried
and the walking wounded.
Scream, I want to say to the rescue workers.
Eyes blank.
Staring at everything and nothing.
Scream your soul.

I want to touch your face,
Hold your mud-crusted hand.
You look into my eyes, holding tight
to my insides.
Your mouth almost smiles.
Energy low.
I smile for you.
Slowly, we pass each other and move
into the quiet thumping of the night.[3]

In "Someone to Fill My Shoes" (*Nursing Spectrum*, 6/3/02), Janet Stevens, the Resource Manager/Clinical Educator for the Nursing Education Department at Good Samaritan Hospital Medical Center in West Islip, NY, wrote about how she found herself reflecting on what being a nurse meant to her when her daughter asked her, "What's the best part of being a nurse, Mommy?" What she said in this article reflects the essence of nursing. Stevens wrote:

". . . It (nursing) is an investment in my patients' lives. I make a difference every day—touching hearts and inspiring souls. This has been my passion for almost two decades. I am an ambassador of hope. I'm not famous and certainly not someone who brings home a six-digit yearly income. But the gifts of being a nurse are almost intangible. It's not measurable. Nursing has made me a better person, more patient, more understanding, and forgiving. I am in awe of the power of the human spirit. I appreciate the fragility of life and remind people to tell those who are precious to them how much they are loved. The World Trade Center's victims and their families gave us all this lesson. I'm reminded of this lesson every day. I am challenged to use leadership skills and motivated to connect with mentors and those they mentor. I nurture. I heal. . . . I get back so much more than I give. I am so blessed."[4]

THE NURSE-PATIENT CARING EQUATION

A concern that has become heightened among many people, nurses included, in this post-9/11 world is a desire to ensure that the quality of one's personal life is not eroded or invaded by the intensity of the work one does. This is an old story and an eternal conflict for nurses that, left unattended, leads to stress and burnout, and eventually the diminishment of quality in the care they are able to give patients. In the wake of September 11th, and during what is predicted to be one of the most profound nursing shortages ever, nurses can no longer afford to ignore this issue, lest society depletes its already scarce nursing personnel resources. One way to understand what is required to meet this challenge is to see the nurse-patient relationship as a kind of math equation, which like all math equations requires balancing. This means that equal attention to both sides of the equation, the nurse and the patient, must occur if both are to benefit from the relationship. When the nurse attends to his or her own needs with the same degree of priority and focus as to the needs of the patient, balance can be achieved. This may never occur simultaneously, nor should it since the nurse-patient relation is not a reciprocal one; but it must occur eventually. To think that the nurse only exists for the benefit of the patient is not only naïve; it has the potential to result in marginal care for the patient, while increasing the likelihood of stress and burnout for the nurse. Or, said differently, there is no real quality in patient care without "nurse care" as well.

Who cares for the nurse is an important question. It would seem that healthcare organizations that want to ensure the quality care they say they want for their patients would be sure that nurses had good work environments, safe staffing ratios, adequate meal breaks, and so on. In the unfortunate absence of these essential work standards in far too many environments, it is left up to each individual nurse to balance the equation for himself or herself. Ignoring the need for this risks the stress and burnout that has long haunted the nursing profession. As a professional, it is up to you to take seriously your individual responsibility to balance the nurse-patient equation. Do this, and you go a long way to ensuring not only quality care for the patient, but professional satisfaction as well, with the added benefit of preventing burnout. See Chapter 16, "The Resilient Nurse: Self-Care Strategies," for self-care and burnout prevention strategies.

MAGNET STATUS ORGANIZATIONS

Healthcare organizations that take responsibility to effectively balance this nurse-patient-care equation are frequently those who have been granted the prestigious Magnet status by the American Nurses Credentialing Center (ANCC), an arm of the American Nurses Association whose mission is to promote excellence in nursing and healthcare globally through credentialing programs and related services. Just as nurses who want to achieve a standard of excellence in their nursing practice can seek ANCC certification, so can organizations. In 2001, 20 organizations (an unprecedented number) qualified for and were granted Magnet status. Currently, over 50 Magnet organizations exist (see the appendix for a current list). These are certainly places from which to seek employment when at all possible. (An alternative might be to use the characteristics of Magnet organizations as a guide to evaluate your potential employers). ANCC's *Credentialing News* described what these excellence-focused Magnet organizations have in common:

- 100 percent of the chief nurse executives at Magnet facilities hold graduate or higher degrees.

- 97 percent of all Magnet organizations have affiliations with schools of nursing, and 91 percent are affiliated with allied health programs.

- 92 percent of the staff at Magnet hospitals attend at least one continuing-education program each year.

- 83 percent of all Magnet facilities have affiliations with schools of medicine.

- 63 percent of all applicants receive Magnet designation.

- 57 percent of nurses who serve in leadership positions at Magnet organizations have at least one graduate degree, 36 percent are advanced practice nurses, and 21 percent are certified.

- 27.5 percent of nurses providing direct care at Magnet hospitals are certified.

- 19 percent of Magnet organizations are organized for collective bargaining purposes.

- The average turnover rate of all Magnet hospitals is 11.5 percent.

- The average vacancy rate among all Magnet hospitals is 8.19 percent.

- The average length of employment among registered nurses at Magnet organizations is 8.83 years.

- The average number of licensed beds among all Magnet organizations is 487; the range is between 100–1,951 licensed beds.

- The average hours per patient day are 10.04 hours across the entire nursing department.

Credentialing News went on to summarize the importance of this data as follows:

"This and other data suggest that Magnet-designated hospitals have outcomes that are positive for patients, nurses, and employers. For patients, lower Medicare mortality rates for patients with AIDS have been seen, as well as shorter lengths of stay, decreased utilization of critical care beds, and increased patient satisfaction. For nurses, satisfaction is increased, as is R.N. skill mix, perception of productivity, and perceived ability to give high-quality care. For employers, there appears to be a lower incidence of needlestick injuries, and nurse burnout rate, as well as an enhanced ability to recruit and retain nurses. Finally, JCAHO (Joint Commission on Accreditation of Healthcare Organizations) scores among Magnet organizations are higher."[5]

The positive influence organizations with Magnet designation have on the welfare of the patient and nurse alike, and how this has the potential to ease the nursing shortage was described in *Report*, the official newsletter of the New York State Nurses Organization (June 2002), which stated that these facilities:

- Respect nursing professionals' knowledge in the development of policies

- Included direct-care nurses on the nurse practice committees that establish staffing plans based on patient acuity and need

- Do not penalize or intimidate nurses who question policies or work to change practices that negatively affect patient care

- Do not force nurses to work overtime to fill gaps in staffing schedules[6]

While seeking employment in a Magnet status organization is a career strategy that can go a long way to ensuring that the nursing practice environment you choose supports *both* your professional and your personal needs, it cannot be the only strategy, since there are not yet enough of them. Perhaps stated more accurately, not enough healthcare organizations have awoken to this 21st-century workplace necessity that benefits patient and nurse alike.

MEETING YOUR PROFESSIONAL AND PERSONAL NEEDS

It may very well be up to *you* to ensure a viable and healthy work environment for yourself. The capacity for this kind of proactivity is one of the hallmark characteristics of the nurse practicing during these early years of the 21st century. Consider the advice of Gloria Steinem, who asserts that actions taken by the individual are as essential as those taken by organizations. In her book, *Revolution from Within, A Book of Self-Esteem,* Steinem said that two revolutions were needed if both society *and* the individual were to achieve egalitarian wholeness and equal opportunity. The first revolution was the one she has led since the 1960s against sexual and racial barriers using social and political action. Her book connects that *outer* revolution to a necessary *inner* revolution of spirit and consciousness. She had initially believed that inner change was not necessary for societal change to occur. She became suspicious, however, that something was missing when she encountered women with too little self-esteem to take advantage of "hard won, if still incomplete, opportunities, and too many (though not only) men who were addicted to authority and control as the only proof of their value." Both, she said, lacked faith in a unique self: that "core" self-esteem without which no amount of situational self-esteem can be enough.

She encourages a persistent, consistent focus and an awareness on two fronts: the individual *and* the collective; the personal *and* the professional. In nursing, that translates into an awareness of yourself as a nurse, *as well as* the organization for which you work; of your individual nursing practice *and* the nursing profession to which you belong.

One without the other dilutes the effect of both. What this means for the nurse who wants personal *and* professional well-being (which translates to burnout protection) is clear: support, work towards, facilitate, and fight for organizational change, *but don't wait for it!* This is a good example of coping with simultaneous realities, another characteristic of the 21st-century nurse: know what you need to take care of yourself (inner awareness), even if the organization (outer awareness) has not provided for it, or worse, creates obstacles when you attempt to do it.

For example, what can you do, or, what are you *willing* to do to ensure that you have adequate nutrition, hydration, and rest when working a 10-hour shift, even if the meal breaks usually are not taken because the workload is too great? Reflect on how you generally respond (or how you imagine yourself responding) as you read what follows.

THE BALANCING ACT

Being routinely unable to meet one's basic needs, as described in the dilemma above could potentially be seen as a disruption in homeostatic balance, in the status quo of one's life, oftentimes evoking a crisis, depending on your response to it and support during it. A crisis is a turning point in which there is the potential for danger as well as opportunity. Interestingly, in the Chinese language, which is written in symbols, the symbol for the word *crisis* is translated to mean both danger *and* opportunity.

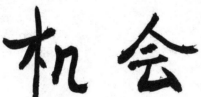

Crisis = Danger + Opportunity

A crisis is a kind of wake-up call, a call to action, if you will. Depending on the action you take or don't take you will either:

Thrive and grow, personally and/or professionally; learn something from the situation

Survive, stay the same, possibly stagnate

Collapse, possibly regress or retreat

What will influence which of these outcomes occurs is your ability to apply the balancing features described below to your situation, as well as how you answer the questions that accompany them. As you read what follows, consider your actual or imagined responses to the dilemma described above.

BALANCING FEATURES ASSOCIATED WITH A CRISIS	QUESTIONS ON WHICH TO REFLECT
1. Accurately perceiving the meaning and impact of the situation	1. Do you see the situation as a threat or a challenge?
2. Establishing and using support systems comprised of people and knowledge	2. Do you have (or can you find) people who can guide you, teach you, and advise you, to whom you can talk and be heard?
3. Utilizing coping strategies effectively to mediate the stress that typically accompanies a crisis	3. Do you have routines, rituals, and habits already in place that are known to lower your stress, or are you able to learn them? Examples include exercise, assertiveness skills, communicating when angry, meditation, and so on.

THRIVING ON CHANGE

While 21st-century nurses are certainly not immune from being bewildered, exasperated, and stressed by changes in the status quo, even if this should evoke a crisis, what makes them *thrivers* rather than *survivors* or *victims* is their perception of the situation as a challenge and the opportunity they see in it for personal and/or professional growth. They are able to navigate through the difficulties that change brings and come out winners, often bringing others along with them.

Another way to envision how this 21st-century nurse functions is to imagine yourself in a boat with other people, rowing down a river, when suddenly the water becomes turbulent and foamy, rocking the boat and the people in it and skirting the choppy, uneven surfaces of half-hidden rocks and boulders. You might be aware that this kind of water is called *whitewater* and the challenging sport associated with it is called *whitewater rafting. Permanent whitewater* is a term used by Jane Schuman in her article, "Navigating the Whitewaters of Change," as a metaphor to describe the permanent conditions of continuous, accelerated change that typified the 1990s and that have become a well-known companion to everyone's life today. Schuman described three different responses to this experience. Which most closely resembles you?

The Victim: You expect the worst and are sure that the danger you imagine just around the next bend will do you in. You are reactive rather than proactive. You spend a lot of time gripping the sides of the raft with white-knuckled terror, blaming and criticizing those trying to steer the boat. You fall into the water, requiring others to divide their attention between steering the boat and rescuing you.

The Survivor: You have your life jacket buttoned securely and will stay afloat, but believe you are only along for the ride and have no choice about the direction of the boat or power to influence anything in the situation. Although you stay safely in the boat, you use all your energy holding on and contribute nothing to guiding the boat to safe waters.

The Navigator: You see this unanticipated situation as a challenge. You are scared at times but get through the swelling currents by developing new skills and retooling old ones. Your confidence grows in proportion to your ability to work with those who are doing the steering. You save the Victim when she falls into the water and reassure the Survivor, whose anxiety is distracting those steering the boat.

It is not so much the intensity of the change that determines whether or not you become a navigator in any particular situation, but rather the degree of control you believe you have over the shape and direction of your predicament. Even though navigators find themselves pessimistic at times (seeing the glass half empty), it is their capacity to *recognize their state of mind and shift to the half-filled nature of the glass* that distinguishes them from the victim or the survivor.

The following profiles describe the experiences of three newly hired direct care nurses who have just completed orientation to the cardiac care center and are all faced with the same dilemma. They are working ten-hour shifts and discover that while meal breaks are assigned by the nurse manager, they are rarely taken by the staff who cite the nurse-patient ratio and patient acuity as too high to permit adequate break time. Which description most closely resembles how you might respond to the situation?

Profile of a Victim: Vicky

Although it is not her preference, Vicky feels obliged to do what others do, and takes no meal breaks. She gulps glasses of water when she can and has learned to ignore the hunger pangs she feels toward the middle of her shift. She has developed headaches but does not connect them to her lowered blood glucose level or need for nutrition. She's also not sleeping as well as she used to.

She finds herself wondering why there is such a mental and physical frenzy among nurses in this new work environment, remembering that in the cardiac care center she just came from, meal breaks were routinely taken even though they had just as few nurses and just as many sick patients. She left that job because she felt harassed by a coworker who complained to the nurse manager that her change of shift reports were too long. She felt too intimidated to confront this coworker or seek assistance from the nurse manager. She had wondered about finding someone to talk to about all this but couldn't figure out how to go about it. She still wonders why her thoroughness was so misunderstood.

Seeing the problems she is in for at this new job, she begins to blame herself for leaving her last job, even though it felt like the right decision at the time. She feels preoccupied, sometimes depressed. She thinks she is powerless to react differently and doesn't see a way out of her situation. She is rarely aware that the needs and preferences of other people almost always take precedence over her own, and when she is aware, she doesn't know what to do about it. She finds herself wondering if nursing was a good career choice after all.

Profile of a Survivor: Sam

Sam usually takes his meal breaks but spends them complaining and being angry because it is so difficult to do so. He is very critical of the nurse manager's organizational skills and leadership style, and believes that the administrators of the medical center care more about their "bottom line" than the patients or the nurses who take care of them. He calls in sick frequently, telling some of his coworkers that he's entitled to these "mental health days" in exchange for the abuse he has to put up with working under conditions he believes are unfair.

He is assigned to be a preceptor for Tim, a new graduate, and seems unaware of the negative influence his attitude is having on him. He feels it is his moral responsibility to show Tim the "ropes" so he knows how to "play the game." He encourages Tim to think twice in responding to requests from peers for assistance if he wants to leave work on time. He declined to participate when the nurse manager asked him to attend a staff meeting to discuss how to develop a strategy for ensuring that nurses got their meal breaks, telling a coworker, "Why bother, nothing ever changes around here. Anyway, that's her job, not mine."

Sam waits impatiently for his next long weekend off or his vacation. He frequently talks about "putting in his time" until retirement.

Profile of a Navigator: Nancy

Nancy is new to cardiac care, having spent the first four years out of school on a general medical unit. While she found it very difficult to take meal breaks as a new graduate, she soon linked her afternoon crankiness and mental dullness to not eating lunch. At first she tried having a snack while doing her morning documentation, but soon realized that while she was sharper mentally as a result, she was still irritable. She eventually recognized that a short rest, along with nutrition and hydration, was essential for these long, intense workdays. Over a two-week period, she figured out how to organize her day around her patients' needs as well as her own. While not ideal, she now takes two or three 20-minute breaks, on most days, during her 10-hour shift, even though it is far less than what she knows she is entitled to.

She also decided to sign up for a relaxation class offered by the Employee Assistance Program and now alternates visualization with meditation for ten minutes during these breaks, and plans to buy a portable CD player to listen to relaxing music so that the noisy hustle and bustle of the unit is dampened.

During her three-month probationary evaluation with June, the nurse manager, the problem of meal breaks came up and Nancy was surprised to find that June felt as strongly as she did about her staff taking their meal breaks but had given up encouraging them in the face of the resistance she met when she did so. The reasons the staff gave her for ignoring their breaks were varied, including inability to organize their time, having trouble saying no, and problems establishing priorities. June believed that her staff indeed wanted meal breaks but couldn't figure out how to take them. As a result of this discussion, June decided to have a staff meeting to discuss the issue and asked Nancy to share her personal struggles and solutions. Nancy agreed and also volunteered to post a notice about the meeting and to generate interest in it.

Nancy's initial feeling of achievement is being slowly eroded by the peer pressure she is experiencing from Sam, one of her coworkers, which started out as subtle criticism. Recently, he has become generally uncooperative and mysteriously unavailable to cover her patients during her breaks. Unsure how to handle this, she sought the advice of Mary, her preceptor for the first job she had after graduation, and who now is one of her mentors. Mary helped Nancy realize that she would benefit from taking an assertiveness course and told her about one she took and how it helped her deal with the dysfunctional communication patterns that typified some groups of nurses. She was fascinated by the term "horizontal violence" used by Mary to describe how a sense of powerlessness to take action or be heard by those in charge can lead to subtle and overt hostility aimed at one another. She decided to learn more about this after she completed the cardiac care orientation next month.

While Vicky might eventually decide to leave nursing practice, it is likely that Sam's survival skills will enable him to stay, but the degree of professional satisfaction he will have is certainly questionable. The capacity Nancy has to navigate the challenges she faces will go a long way to ensuring a productive and satisfying career, with the additional ability to lead others as well. Nancy's attitude, behavior, and self-awareness is characteristic of what is required of the 21st-century nurse.

CHARACTERISTICS OF THE 21st-CENTURY NURSE

The person who practices nursing in the 21st century requires a commitment to the development and deepening of the personal and professional characteristics described in the following list. As you read this list, use it to determine which characteristics you already have and which you need to develop. This list is not meant to be all-inclusive, but rather, an overview and introduction to additional characteristics you will find in the chapters that follow.

21st-Century Nurses:
- ❏ Recognize the importance of having a B.S.N. or are working toward it
- ❏ Participate in continuing education in traditional as well as online venues
- ❏ Have professional certification at the generalist or specialist level, or at the basic or advanced level

- ❏ Seek professional membership, including the American Nurses Association and other associations or organizations relevant to their nursing practice interests
- ❏ Possess broad cross-training in nursing skills and competencies
- ❏ Are the Nurse CEOs of their self-owned nursing practice called *You, Inc.,* considering themselves self-employed even if they work for others
- ❏ Know how to maintain loyalty to self, while simultaneously committing to the mission of the organization that is currently employing them
- ❏ Can articulate the vision, mission, and values that drive their nursing practice
- ❏ Find mentors and mentor others
- ❏ Demonstrate leadership and are self-starters
- ❏ Are self-directed as well as team-oriented
- ❏ Utilize proactive behaviors and assertive communication styles
- ❏ Are flexible and creative thinkers
- ❏ Are willing to take informed risks and learn from their mistakes
- ❏ Take self-care skills as seriously as patient-care skills, recognizing that one without the other neutralizes the effectiveness of both
- ❏ Expect changes significant enough to alter their work or personal lives about every six months
- ❏ Know their limits and are not afraid of using the word "no"
- ❏ Never abdicate personal responsibility for themselves
- ❏ Are technologically proficient, computer literate, and Internet savvy
- ❏ Are avid personal and professional networkers in traditional and online venues

Add additional characteristics important to you but not mentioned in the space provided below:

☐ _____

☐ _____

☐ _____

☐ _____

☐ _____

YOUR THREE-LEGGED STOOL OF NURSING SUCCESS

To succeed as a 21ˢᵗ-century nurse means to control the direction and the quality of your nursing practice by attending to these three inextricably linked skill-sets:

- Professional and clinical skills
- Career management skills
- Self-care skills

You can envision these companionate skill-sets as three distinct but interrelated legs of a three-legged stool. Imagine what would happen if one or more of these legs were unevenly matched to the others. It would certainly wobble and fail to support anyone using it. Likewise, neglecting one or more of these legs representing the tripartite whole of your nursing practice is a prescription for the lack of balance typically responsible for stress and burnout.

SKILL SETS	EXAMPLES
Professional and clinical skills	Delegating Assessing respiratory patterns
Career management skills	Writing a resume Networking
Self-care skills	Assertiveness Stress management

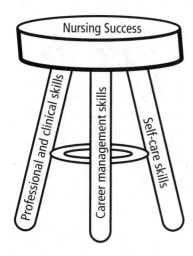

Your nursing education, whether basic, graduate, or continuing, supports the professional/clinical leg of this three-legged stool. Career seminars and resources such as this book or Internet sites support the career management leg. Learning stress management skills, attending personal development seminars, and even psychotherapy are ways to ensure that the third leg, self-care, reflects the same strength as the others. Chapter 16, "The Resilient Nurse: Self-Care Strategies," will deepen this discussion and provide you with opportunities to explore what this means to your career as a nurse, and the quality of your life as a whole.

NURSES: THE PEOPLE IN THE PARENTHESES

We have become what psychologist and human potential expert Jean Houston calls "the people in the parentheses," those people suspended between what was and what will be as the healthcare industry and the nursing profession continue to position and reposition themselves to meet the needs of patients and workers alike. We belong to the generation of nurses bridging the gap between old and new, past and future, now and to be. Life within the parentheses is challenging and sometimes threatening to our professional and personal wholeness, integrity, and well-being as we struggle to maintain our footing in a constantly changing world.

John Naisbitt, author of *Megatrends: Ten New Directions Transforming Our Lives*, echoes this by saying:

> "We are living in the time of the parentheses, the time between eras. Those who are willing to handle the ambiguity of this in-between period and to anticipate the new era will be a quantum leap ahead of those who hold on to the past. The time of the parentheses is a time of change and questioning. Although the time between eras is uncertain, it is a great and yeasty time, filled with opportunity. If we can learn to make uncertainty our friend, we can achieve much more than in stable eras. In stable eras, everything has a name and everything knows its place and we can leverage very little. But in the time of the parentheses we have extraordinary leverage and influence, individually, professionally, institutionally, if we can get a clear sense, a clear conception, a clear vision, of the road ahead. My God, what a fantastic time to be alive!"[7]

And, what a fantastic time to be a nurse!

The World of Nursing Practice

Nursing is a knowledge-based profession, a significant fact that is often not fully understood nor appreciated. The nurse's ability to be a critical thinker and to use knowledge in the delivery of nursing care is essential to the well-being of those for whom nurses care. The basis for the scientific practice of nursing includes nursing science, the biomedical, physical, economic, behavioral, and social sciences, and ethics and philosophy. Nurses are concerned with human experience and responses to birth, health, illness, and death. Nurses care for individuals, families, communities, and populations. In her book *Life Support*, Suzanne Gordon observes:

> "Although nurses help us to live and die, in the public depiction of healthcare, patients seem to emerge from hospitals without ever having benefited from their assistance. Whether patients are treated in an emergency room in a few short hours, or on a critical care unit for months on end, we seem certain that physicians are responsible for all of the successes—or failures—in our medical system. In fact, we seem to believe that they are responsible not only for all of the curing, but for much of the caring. Nurses, on the other hand, remain shadowy figures moving mysteriously in the background . . . In our high-tech medical system, nurses are the ones who care for the body and the soul . . . nurses are often closer to patients' needs and wishes than physicians . . . they spend far more time with patients and know them better."[1]

DEFINING NURSING PRACTICE

There are a variety of definitions of nursing practice. Florence Nightingale proposed that nursing practice involved being in "charge of the personal health of somebody . . . and what nursing has to do . . . is to put the patient in the best condition for nature to act upon him."[2] According to Virginia Henderson, nursing practice was "to assist the individual, sick or well, in the performance of those activities contributing to health or its recovery (or to a peaceful death) that he would perform unaided if he had the necessary strength, will, or knowledge, and to do this in such a way as to help him gain independence as rapidly as possible."[3] In many state nurse practice acts, the practice of professional nursing is defined as the diagnosis and treatment of human responses to actual or potential health problems. The American Nurses Association (ANA) proposes that there are four essential features inherent in any definition of contemporary nursing practice:

- Attention to the full range of human experiences and responses to health and illness without restriction to a problem-focused orientation
- Integration of objective data with knowledge gained from an understanding of the individual, family, community, or population's subjective experience
- Application of scientific knowledge to the processes of diagnosis and treatment
- Provision of a caring relationship that facilitates health and healing[4]

THE LEGAL FOUNDATIONS OF NURSING PRACTICE

All registered professional nurses (R.N.s) are independent practitioners of the profession. Licensed practical nurses (L.P.N.s) are dependent practitioners of nursing and deliver nursing care under the direction or supervision of an R.N. or otherwise authorized healthcare practitioner. The practice of nursing is authorized by the licensure bodies of the states and directed by professional nursing organizations. Nurses are held accountable to the laws, regulations, and rules of the licensing authority and the standards and ethics of the profession as promulgated by the various nursing groups. It is a professional responsibility of a nurse to be a lifelong learner and to be knowledgeable of the legal and professional expectations associated with the practice of the profession. This includes applicable state laws and regulations governing nursing practice and the delivery of healthcare services.

In 2003, the American Nurses Association (ANA) published *Nursing's Social Policy Statement (Second Edition)* in which is expressed the social contract that exists between nursing and society. In it is noted that the relationship between a nurse and a patient (individual, family, community, population) involves a "full and active participation of the patient and the nurse in the plan of care within the context of the values and beliefs of the patient and the nurse." There are four basic values and assumptions on which this statement is predicated:

- Humans manifest an essential unity of mind, body, and spirit.
- Human experience is contextually and culturally defined.
- Health and illness are human experiences.
- The presence of illness does not preclude health, nor does optimal health preclude illness.[5]

In the United States, the legal authorization for nursing practice is contained in the Nurse Practice Acts of the states, and in other countries in the country's or province's applicable laws. Such acts can be general in the description of nursing practice or be very specific, listing authorized tasks or acts. Professional licensure has been established to protect the public from harm and to authorize the practice of a profession. States usually require a demonstration of attaining and successfully completing a specific education, verification of minimal competency by passing the national nursing licensure examination (NCLEX-RN® exam), and evidence of good moral character. Licensure is a privilege, not a right. Once a nurse is authorized to practice the profession of nursing, the state expects that in all aspects of the nurse's life that there will be an awareness of this privilege and that the nurse will remain personally committed to meeting any new educational requirements, maintaining appropriate competence in practice, and not engaging in any acts of professional misconduct such as gross incompetence, negligence, fraud, conviction of a felony or misdemeanor, practicing while impaired, or specific unprofessional conduct acts as defined by the state (e.g., abusing a patient, failure to appropriately document, revealing personally identifiable information or facts about a patient, and inappropriately delegating professional acts).

In addition to the various state nurse practice acts, there are other state and federal laws that can impact upon a professional nursing practice. These include the conditions of participation of Medicare and Medicaid, the Emergency Medical Treatment and Active Labor Act (EMTALA), and various public health and/or state laws that describe how healthcare facilities (hospitals, nursing homes, diagnostic and treatment centers, ambulatory/outpatient centers, home care agencies, hospices, assisted living facilities) must function in any specific jurisdiction. In addition, professional practice can be impacted by the availability or lack of reimbursement for nursing services and by the credentialing requirements of such groups as the federal Education Department, Health and Human Services, the Center for Medicare and Medicaid (CMS), the Joint Commission for Accreditation of Healthcare Organizations (JCAHO), and state or local health and education departments.

THE ETHICS OF NURSING

Nursing practice is based on an ethical tradition. ANA's *Code of Ethics for Nurses* explicitly expresses the primary goals, values, and obligations of the profession. The *Code* has two components—the nine provisions and the accompanying interpretative statements. The latter explain in greater detail each of the provisions and place the provision in the context of current nursing practice. The nine provisions include:

- The nurse, in all professional relationships, practices with compassion and respect for the inherent dignity, worth, and uniqueness of every individual, unrestricted by considerations of social or economic status, personal attributes, or the nature of health problems.
- The nurse's primary commitment is to the patient, whether an individual, family, group, or community.
- The nurse promotes, advocates for, and strives to protect the health, safety, and rights of the patient.
- The nurse is responsible and accountable for individual nursing practice and determines appropriate delegation of tasks consistent with the nurse's obligation to provide optimum patient care.
- The nurse owes the same duties to self as to others, including the responsibility to preserve integrity and safety, to maintain competence, and to continue personal and professional growth.
- The nurse participates in establishing, maintaining, and improving healthcare environments and conditions of employment conducive to the provision of quality healthcare and consistent with the values of the profession through individual and collective action.
- The nurse participates in the advancement of the profession through contributions to practice, education, administration, and knowledge development.

- The nurse collaborates with other health professionals and the public in promoting community, national, and international efforts to meet health needs.
- The profession of nursing, as represented by associations and their members, is responsible for articulating nursing values, for maintaining the integrity of the profession and its practice, and for shaping social policy.

STANDARDS OF NURSING PRACTICE

ANA in collaboration with the national specialty nursing organizations has established standards of nursing practice for both generic and specialty nursing practice. The various standards describe a competent level of nursing care; reflect the values and priorities of the profession; provide direction for professional practice; and form a basis of accountability for all nurses regardless of practice setting. ANA's *Nursing: Scope and Standards of Practice* focuses on the processes of providing care (Standards of Care) and performing professional role activities (Standards of Professional Performance). The Standards of Practice describe a competent level of nursing care based on a critical thinking model known as the nursing process and include: assessment, diagnosis, outcome identification, planning, implementation, and evaluation. The Standards of Professional Performance describe a competent level of behavior in the professional nursing role and include: quality of care, performance appraisal, education, collegiality, ethics, collaboration, research, resource utilization, and leadership. Each standard consists of a standard statement (e.g., assessment—the nurse collects patient health data) and various measurement criteria (e.g., data collection involves the patient, family, and other healthcare providers as appropriate) for meeting the standard. These criteria are essential indicators of professional nursing practice and all identified measurement criteria must be met in order for the standard to be met.

In addition, nurses can be held to local standards of nursing practice to describe what a reasonable and prudent nurse is expected to do. These local standards are usually the policies and procedures of the healthcare facility in which the nurse is employed. Employers' policies are considered essentially a permit to practice nursing in that facility. These policies can limit the R.N.'s legal scope of practice, but they cannot expand it. For instance, in most states it is considered within the scope of practice of an R.N. to start an IV, but facilities do not have to let all R.N.s perform this procedure. The employer's policies and procedures must be in compliance with the state's Nurse

Practice Act and any other laws, regulations, or rules that govern practice; they should reflect the professional standards of practice and address the expected ethical behavior.[6]

NURSES' RIGHTS AND RESPONSIBILITIES

While the laws and regulations, standards of nursing practice, and the *Code of Ethics for Nurses* collectively address nurses' rights, obligations, and responsibilities, nurses can be puzzled regarding their rights and responsibilities. The New York State Nurses Association, in a paper discussing rights and responsibilities, defined a right as a just claim to something to which one is entitled, a prerogative, an entitlement, a political statement, or a legal declaration. In addition, a responsibility was defined as a trust or duty owed by one individual to another. There are three types of rights: fundamental human rights; legal rights, including those inherent in practice acts; and professional rights, such as the right to provide nursing care, the right to independent nursing practice judgment, the right to the necessary knowledge to safely practice, the right to ensure safe care environments, the right to advocate for the patient, the right to control the practice environment, the right to protest or refuse an unsafe practice assignment with the understanding of the risks and consequences involved, the right to proper professional economic compensation, and so on.

It is important to recognize that rights regardless of the type are not absolutes and choosing the "greater good" in professional practice involves risk-taking and may have employment, legal, ethical, or disciplinary consequences. According to ANA, the intrinsic linking of nurses' rights to professional responsibility can lead to frustration, a feeling of powerlessness and a sense of inadequacy.[7] Dr. Claire Fagin has noted that nurses develop rights by having an image of themselves as being worthy of such rights, by sharing information about the profession and the work of nurses, through concerted advocacy, and by doing something for society that society values—not by being victims or pleading. The New York State Nurses Association has noted that:

> "Rights and responsibilities are segments of a single professional practice continuum. It is only through collective action that nurses can truly fulfill the responsibilities of nursing practice. As professional nurses, we will move forward learning the critical lessons of similar rights movements that strength and power are greater when pursued by a united group moving forward together."[8]

NURSING PRACTICE AND THE NURSING SHORTAGE

It is difficult to address nursing practice in this century without acknowledging the "elephant in the living room"—the national and global nursing shortage and its current and potential impact. In its materials, the ANA differentiates between a staffing shortage and a nursing shortage. A staffing shortage is a present-day concern and reflects "an insufficient number, mix, and/or experience of registered nurses and ancillary staff to safely care for the individual and aggregate needs of a specific patient population over a specific period of time." The nursing shortage is a more long-term concern and reflects "more of an economic perspective as the demand and need for registered nurses' services is greater than the supply of registered nurses who are qualified, available, and willing to work." (*Memo for CMA Executive Directors on Nursing's Agenda for the Future*, ANA, 2002).[9] Throughout the 20th century there were cyclical periods identified as nursing shortages. Some of the quick fixes that were used to alleviate the various shortages included: changes in work hours, financial bonuses for employment, increased wages, scholarships and grants to support education, attracting "second careerists" into the profession, foreign nurse recruitment, increased utilization of unlicensed assistive personnel, pay differentials and incentives for different shift work and specialty nursing, changes in practice modalities, and more attention to the contributions of the nursing staff by the facilities and employers. However, the burdens associated with the work environment and the overall structure of the healthcare system in our nation was never adequately addressed.

According to Peter Buerhaus, a nurse researcher, the R.N. workforce is aging in the near term and shrinking in the longer term (*News & Views*, Rhode Island Nurses' Association, 2000). He provides some cautionary statistics:

- The average age of employed R.N.s increased more than twice as fast as all other occupations in the U.S. workforce in the past 15 years.

- More than 60 percent of working R.N.s are older than 40; by 2010, more than 40 percent of the R.N. workforce will be older than 50.

- Between 2010 and 2020, many R.N.s will start to retire with the largest working group of R.N.s being between 50 and 60; this coincides with many of the nation's baby boomers turning 65 and entering the Medicare system.[10]

In addition, the 2000 *National Sample Survey of Registered Nurses* (NSSRN) provided a wealth of information about the R.N. workforce including:

- The average amount of time spent by R.N.s on doing nondirect patient care was 37 percent.

- Increasing numbers of R.N.s—18.3 percent of the national R.N. workforce—are choosing not to work in nursing.
- Of nurses employed outside of nursing, 20 percent cite concern for safety in the healthcare environment as a reason for having another occupation.
- Of R.N.s employed in a variety of nursing positions, 19.8 percent are either moderately or extremely dissatisfied with their positions.

The federal Bureau of Labor Statistics identifies nursing as one of the ten occupations projected to have the largest amount of openings in the next decade. There are 2.7 million nurses constituting the nation's largest healthcare profession. Currently, there are a reported 126,000 R.N. vacancies in the nation. By 2020, an article in JONA projects an estimated 400,000 R.N. vacancies with a lack of 650,000 baccalaureate-prepared nurses nationwide.[11] This shortage will impact on all healthcare settings, not just hospitals.

PROJECTED NURSING SHORTAGE: 2001–2020

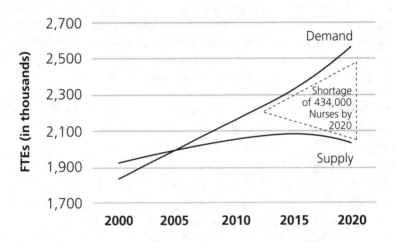

Source: Johnson & Johnson, The Campaign for Nursing's Future (Buerhaus, et al., JAMA, June 2000).

In April 2002, the Robert Wood Johnson Foundation (RWJ) released its report *Health Care's Human Crisis: the American Nursing Shortage*. Dr. Steven Schroder, RWJ President and CEO, comments that:

> "While we haven't seen a consumer backlash about the nursing crisis . . . there is more dissatisfaction out there than we are willing to acknowledge

. . . consumers don't perceive the nursing shortage as an abstraction or a problem for hospital human resources departments to handle, but are already feeling its detrimental effect on the quality of care that they receive at the bedside. We must act soon."

Of particular concern to the researchers is the fact that the nursing shortage endangers quality of care, places patients at risk, and could undermine the entire American healthcare industry. The report unequivocally states that the current nursing shortage will extend well into the 21st century and is driven by a broader and different set of factors than the shortages that were experienced in the last century. These factors are identified as:

- The reality of an aging population, especially the 80 million baby boomers
- Fewer younger people entering the workforce, creating a "war for talent"
- The physical demands of nursing practice preventing most nurses from working past their mid-50s
- The lack of racial and ethnic diversity in the nursing workforce
- Due to the opportunities created by the women's rights movement, women have chosen other professions or work over nursing and not enough men have entered the profession to compensate for this change
- The perception by younger workers such as those in Generation X that nursing is unappealing
- Increased consumer activism
- A ballooning healthcare system with nursing lacking the authority to create and sustain change

The report recommends a "reenvisioning of the nursing profession itself, so that it can emerge from this crisis stronger and in equal partnership with the profession of medicine" to be accomplished by the creation of a National Forum to Advance Nursing. Involved in the Forum would be: nurses and nursing profession leaders, educators, healthcare industry leaders, labor unions, government, and the various national nursing and healthcare organizations and consumers. The Forum would focus its efforts on the following areas:

- Creating new nursing models and advancing nursing's contributions to healthcare outcomes and consumer satisfaction
- Reinventing nursing education and work environments to appeal to and address the needs and values of a new generation of nurses

- Establishing a national nursing workforce measurement and data collection system
- Creating a clearinghouse of effective strategies to advance cultural change within the nursing profession[12]

In a medical newsletter recently, there was a commentary by a physician, Michael Greenberg, M.D. In it he observed that:

"Nurses are full-fledged partners in the healthcare equation, offering not only their compassionate perspective but also their eyes, ears and hearts . . . they have prevented me from doing or saying something foolish, or worse, harming a patient . . . Nurses are a priceless healthcare resource that is not being renewed or protected."[13]

WHAT THIS MEANS TO YOUR NURSING PRACTICE

Control of your own nursing practice is essential. It is important for nurses to choose to work in environments that understand, value, and support each nurse's practice. As nursing practice evolves in the 21st century and the global nursing shortage is addressed, nurses need to carefully and systematically assess the complex dynamics that influence the ability to practice in any healthcare setting. This should begin with an honest and clear assessment of what is important to your practice. A state nurses association has suggested that information be obtained related to the following:

- The actual clinical practice that will be expected
- The availability of clinical preceptors
- Utilization of technical supports (computer systems, pharmacy dispersal, laboratory access)
- The availability of ancillary support (nursing assistants, housekeeping, dietary, transportation, clerical)
- Access to staff development and education
- Salaries and benefits
- Creative staffing and scheduling
- Contact with and responsiveness of nursing management[14]

One way of finding a supportive practice environment is to seek to practice in a facility that has been granted Magnet hospital status by the American Nurses Credentialing Center (ANCC), as discussed in Chapter 1. This program is based on a 1983 study by the American Academy of Nursing that sought to identify the characteristics of hospitals that were able to successfully attract and retain professional nurses even in times of shortage. The authors noted that:

> ". . . the large number of instances in which the word 'listen' is used by both the directors and the staff nurses . . . Typical of the responses given by directors of nursing is this statement: 'Listen to the staff . . . the best consultants are on your own staff'. Staff nurses tend to say much the same thing . . . 'listen to the patient contact people, they know what they are talking about' . . . it is the clear implication that the listening will be done well—that careful consideration is given to what is being said and the intent of utilizing the ideas set forth . . . ."[15]

As discussed in other sections of this book, it is essential that all nurses have a clear direction for their own professional growth and when changes need to be made in how and where they choose to practice nursing. This means making choices about educational and clinical advancement and specialty certification. Educational choices can include continuing-education courses, master's or doctoral work, while clinical advancement can include deciding to become an advanced practice registered nurse (A.P.R.N.) such as a nurse practitioner, clinical nurse specialist, nurse anesthetist, or nurse midwife and/or deciding to specialize in a particular field of nursing. The designation A.P.R.N. is generally becoming recognized within the profession as a general term to describe these four nursing categories. In some states the title advanced practice registered nurse (A.P.R.N.) or advanced practice nurse (A.P.N.) has been incorporated in the nurse practice act as a legal title. ANA has developed a scope of practice and standards of practice for A.P.R.N.s; full descriptions of these practices are given in Chapter 3, "The State of Nursing Education."

Certification in a clinical (e.g., pediatrics, medical-surgical, psychiatric-mental health) or role (e.g., administrator, informatics, staff development) specialty is a process that professional nurses use to demonstrate proficiency and expertise. Certification generally requires graduation from an accredited/approved educational program in the specialty; recommendations from professional colleagues and satisfactory completion of a certification examination that can be administered by the American Nurses Credentialing Center or a specialty nursing organization.

Staffing

It is quite clear that the nursing workplace environment must be improved in order to reduce the burden on the currently practicing nurses, to provide an incentive for individuals to enter or return to nursing, and to encourage nurses to stay active in the profession for longer periods. This includes the establishment of adequate and appropriate safe staffing. Recently, there has been interest in legislatively mandating specific staffing ratios. The problem with this type of solution is that the established ratio instead of being a minimum number will more than likely become the maximum staffing level. Ratios also do not address the differences in the various healthcare facilities regarding patient acuity or encourage responding to shift-to-shift or unit-to-unit differences in staffing needs. It would be better to consider having the state health authority establish critical elements (e.g., patient acuity, census, skills of the staff, staff mix, geography of the unit, technology) that must be considered in any staffing methodology being used by a healthcare facility and let the facility adapt the formula to its specific needs. The state could review the methodology for appropriateness and hold the facility responsible for meeting the established staffing levels.

Overtime

It is also critical that employers stop relying upon mandatory overtime as a staffing method. In times of real emergencies or unexpected sick calls, many nurses voluntarily offer to work the additional shift. What today's nurses object to is the reliance of the employer to staff a unit by routinely mandating overtime. This type of practice produces a tired, disgruntled, frustrated nurse who in some circumstances may be unsafe. After 16, 18, 20 hours of work, how efficiently can the nurse be expected to be functioning? Nurses also want to be able to meet their responsibilities for their families including child and elder care. It is extremely unfortunate that some employers are threatening nurses with charges of patient abandonment if they do not stay for the mandated overtime. Most states have very specific definitions of what legally constitutes patient abandonment. Nurses should be familiar with their state's rule on this issue and be prepared to formally protest any assignment that will create an unsafe practice situation for themselves and the patients.

Delegating

In today's healthcare environment, nurses are often asked to delegate or assign tasks to other caregivers—other R.N.s, L.P.N.s or unlicensed assistive personnel (U.A.P.s). The differences and distinctions between delegating and assigning differ from state to state. Therefore, all nurses should make sure that they understand what is legally permitted in their states of licensure. Generally, it is illegal for a registered nurse to permit another R.N., an L.P.N. or U.A.P. to perform any task that the R.N. knows the other caregiver is not qualified to perform by reason of licensure, education, or competency. Nurses must develop a clear understanding of what constitutes the protected scope of nursing practice and use this understanding to make appropriate assignments and to ensure that the public receives safe and effective nursing care. Therefore, it is important that R.N.s know the competencies of other R.N.s, the competencies and legal practice of the L.P.N. and the types of tasks that can be performed by a U.A.P.

In 1990, the American Association of Critical Care Nurses (AACN) developed a list of six risk factors that an R.N. could use when evaluating if a U.A.P. could perform a certain task on a particular patient. These risk factors are: potential for harm; condition/stability of the patient; complexity of the task; the level of problem solving or innovation that might be needed; the unpredictability of the outcome; and the level of interaction required with the patient to successfully complete the task. It is an expected professional standard that the R.N. will provide the appropriate levels of direction and supervision when any nursing care is being delivered by a U.A.P.

Malpractice

Nurses are increasingly concerned that the staffing problems in the workplace will result in disciplinary actions, criminal charges, or civil malpractice suits. Malpractice is the type of negligence that occurs when a professional violates a standard of care of the profession. Nursing malpractice occurs when a nurse makes a mistake that harms a patient and the mistake is one that a reasonably careful nurse would not have made in a similar situation. According to a major liability insurance carrier, there are seven main practice categories that can lead to malpractice litigation:

- Nonadherence to basic or fundamental nursing protocol (e.g., administering an unknown medication)
- Failure to recognize signs and symptoms of a medical condition or complications (e.g., inadequate assessment)
- Failure to intervene appropriately (e.g., failure to report changes in a patient's condition)
- Improper performance of psychomotor skills (e.g., nonadherence to principles of asepsis)
- Failure to act as a patient advocate and ensure that competent treatment was received (e.g., acceptance of a passive, "do what you are told" role)

- Inadequate communication between the nurse and the patient, nursing supervisor and/or physician (e.g., failure to listen to and convey an understanding of the patient's complaints and needs)
- Failure to adhere to the nurse's role as a teacher (e.g., lack of teaching about medication management and drug side effects)

In order to decrease the incidence of malpractice charges, it is important for nurses to remember that it is essential to assess the patient on a regular basis and report changes to the M.D., N.P., P.A., and/or nursing supervisor; remember to document and communicate clearly with the patient and the family. It is also prudent for nurses to have their own malpractice insurance. Often nurses rely on the employer's insurance. However, this insurance covers only incidents that occur when one is actually working. Since one is always a nurse, any advice or care that is rendered outside of the employment situation can also result in malpractice claims. While some states have Good Samaritan Laws, one would still have to legally prove that the law applied to the situation being litigated. Malpractice insurance should provide coverage for each claim and aggregate claims; a defendant expense benefit; a personal injury liability; deposition representation; and defense of disciplinary charges.

POLITICAL ACTION

Increasingly nurses are engaging in grassroots legislative activities and political action to promote nursing's agenda for healthcare, to improve workplace conditions and to provide funding for nursing scholarships, grants, and research. ANA successfully lobbied for the passage of the Nurse Reinvestment Act of 2002, which provided monies to boost nursing school enrollments, encourage nurses to return to school for advanced degrees, and support the utilization of the magnet criteria in healthcare facilities.

ANA was particularly disappointed when the Department of Labor rescinded the Ergonomics Program Standards after working two years for its passage. Nurses, as they age, are increasingly concerned about the lack of adequate ergonomic guidelines and rules, especially with the numbers of work-related musculoskeletal injuries that nurses experience. In April 2002, the Department of Labor issued a new ergonomics program. ANA labeled the plan inadequate, as the guidelines would be voluntary and not used as the basis for enforcement. ANA will continue to work with the Congress to achieve passage of comprehensive ergonomics legislation that applies to all healthcare settings.

political action committees (PACs) are one way that individuals and groups can gain access to legislators and other elected officials. PACs endorse and support candidates and officeholders. Through grassroots activities PACs encourage individuals to contact politicians and get nursing's message out. This message can be heard both through financial support and by voting. The democratic process requires the involvement of all citizens and getting nursing's message out requires that nurses learn to share their knowledge and experiences with candidates, legislators, and officeholders.

CHANGING THE FUTURE OF NURSING

Both the staffing and nursing shortages have produced a unique opportunity for nurses, the nursing profession, and all other interested stakeholders once and for all to stop the cyclical nursing shortages. But, one can question whether or not the motivation to change this cycle is present. The healthcare industry in this nation has failed to appreciate that in many healthcare settings, the main commodity that is being provided is nursing care, not medical care. This is not said to diminish the value of the services provided by our physician colleagues, but to emphasize that often most of the care required by patients in hospitals, nursing homes, clinics, home care, and hospices is nursing care. Unfortunately, the healthcare industry, in its convoluted struggles with managed care, cost cutting, changes in reimbursement, onerous regulations, increasing demands of technology, and burdensome documentation, has not been able to construct a workplace environment to successfully support the delivery of nursing care to the satisfaction of both the nurses and the patients and is reluctant to provide adequate compensation for nursing care.

The workplace environment, including improved communication between direct care nurses and nursing management and administration, staffing flexibility and appropriate staffing formulas, no mandatory overtime, adequate compensation, minimizing hazards, and promoting safety, must be addressed to support both retention and recruitment. It is essential to establish the baccalaureate degree as the entry into professional nursing practice or the knowledge needed to support increasingly complex nursing care will be lost. Also needed are increased technological support, reduction of unnecessary and redundant paperwork, recruitment of men and minorities, and improving the media and public's image of nursing.

The nation has for decades struggled with how to develop from the complex healthcare industry a true and functional healthcare system for all that would assure access, quality, and affordable services. In 1993, ANA developed *Nursing's Agenda for*

Health Care Reform. This document declared that the healthcare system was in crisis. The nursing profession called for immediate healthcare reform to include:

- A basic core of essential healthcare services to be available to everyone
- A restructured healthcare system that would focus on the consumers and their health
- Services to be provided in familiar, convenient sites for the public such as schools, workplaces, and homes
- Access to a full range of qualified health professionals
- A shift from the predominant focus on illness and cure to an orientation toward wellness and care[16]

In 2002, ANA announced *Nursing's Agenda for the Future*—an attempt to involve as many nurses as possible in charting the profession's future. Nurses were asked to develop a vision for nursing in 2010. They constructed the following:

> "Nursing is the pivotal healthcare profession, highly valued for its specialized knowledge, skill, and caring in improving the health status of the public and ensuring safe, effective, quality care. The profession mirrors the diverse population it serves and provides leadership to create positive changes in health policy and delivery systems. Individuals choose nursing as a career, and remain in the profession, because of the opportunities for personal and professional growth, supportive work environments, and compensation commensurate with roles and responsibilities."

KNOWLEDGE AND INSPIRED CARING

Nursing and nurses are essential to the delivery of healthcare in this nation. The fact that the profession remains essentially misunderstood should not be viewed as a negative, but as an opportunity to be inspired. Nurses need to be inspired to proclaim nursing's work and identify the beneficial outcomes of our practice. Nurses must be inspired to understand the full scope of nursing practice and to protect it from being diminished. We need to be inspired to accept full responsibility for our own personal lifelong learning and to plan our careers. The career path that will support our practice of the profession of nursing deserves to be inspirationally planned, not allowed to just haphazardly occur. Nurses need to be inspired to remember that the focus of nursing practice is the patient, whether an individual, family, community, or population. Nursing practice is knowledge combined with inspired caring; it will forever remain both an art and a science.

CHAPTER 3

The State of
Nursing Education

Webster's dictionary defines education as follows:

Education: the process of educating

Educating: the development of skill, knowledge, or character

The American Association of Colleges (AACN), in "Nursing Education's Agenda for the 21st Century" says the following about nursing education:

"Nursing education is occurring within the context of rapidly changing technologies and dramatically expanding knowledge."

Daryl Conner, in *Managing at the Speed of Change*, writes:

"The growth of information is occurring so fast that the 'shelf life' of facts and technology has been reduced to almost nothing."[1]

YOUR BELIEFS ABOUT NURSING EDUCATION

Within the context of the three statements above, place a check mark next to the one statement of the following that indicates what you believe about nursing education:

❐ I did my stint in school. It didn't teach me the skills I needed to be a nurse. I learned that from my preceptor. There's no way I'm wasting my time on something like that again. I'm just glad it's over. If this hospital wants me to get more education, let them pay for it and give me the time off to do it. Otherwise, forget it!

❐ I know it's important to keep learning, but honestly, how can I fit it into my schedule? I'm exhausted from my life as it is; how can I think of adding school on top of everything I'm doing? I'm working full time, about to have my third child, and my parents need my attention more these days.

❐ I enjoy learning. There's no way to be an effective nurse today without a solid education to begin with and ongoing learning to keep current. But it's hard to figure out how to do it. I was attending in-service education programs at my hospital until a few months ago when staffing got worse and made it too difficult. So, I've begun to explore the online CE sites and I'm talking to other nurses on my listserv to hear what they are doing.

If your belief about nursing education is reflected in the first response, you might want to reconsider nursing as a career choice since what you learned in nursing school needed updating almost as soon as you learned it. That's the nature of knowledge in the 21st century. (What would you think if your dentist or car mechanic thought this way?)

Most likely, your response was some combination of the second two sets of comments, knowing that education is important and being committed to it, but having difficulty juggling it along with your other responsibilities.

ESSENTIAL TRUTHS ABOUT EDUCATION

A few ideas about education seem important to state. Place a check next to those with which you agree:

❐ *Education is a process*, not an end point. Things change. The faster they change, the more there is to learn.

❐ The goal of education is to *teach you how to learn* about what you need to know, giving you the latest example of how this looks and where you might be using it.

❐ *It is up to you* to ensure that you continue learning when the "next new thing" arrives, whether it is a new piece of technology, or a different procedure, or another conceptual framework to apply in your work as a nurse.

❐ Whether or not your employer provides you with incentives to learn, financial or otherwise, is incidental to ensuring that nursing education remains one of *your professional responsibilities*. While no one would turn down this employment benefit, the absence of it does not let you off the hook, especially since it is a *standard of nursing practice*, often required for license renewal or certification.

❑ Your commitment to nursing education and clinical advancement gives you a *clear direction for your professional growth*, including how and where you choose to practice nursing.

The material in this chapter is designed to give you the information you need to make informed choices about your nursing education, including basic entry level programs, master's level programs, doctoral programs, options for advanced practice, professional certification, and how to ensure your ongoing continuing education. Print and online resources will be mentioned throughout the chapter to help you explore this area of your professional development in greater depth. The resources at the back of this book will give you still further information.

THE NURSING SHORTAGE

As healthcare organizations scramble to find enough nurses to care for an ever-increasing number of more acutely ill patients, colleges and schools of nursing are working hard to recruit and educate the nurses they need. Elsewhere in this book (for example, Chapter 2, "The World of Nursing Practice") you will find discussions about the nursing shortage and its impact on your work as a nurse. Issues about the nursing shortage that are especially relevant to nursing education include (1) faculty shortages and (2) strategies being developed by the nursing education community to recruit and educate more nurses.

The Faculty Shortage

An insufficient and shrinking number of nursing faculty has resulted in the turning away of qualified nursing school applicants, a factor that has influenced the decline in nursing school enrollments and contributed to the national nursing shortage. As the average age of the professional nurse continues to climb, so does the average age of the nursing faculty. The American Association of Colleges of Nursing (AACN, *aacn. nche.edu*) identifies the median age of nurse faculty as 51 years old in 2002, which is anticipated to increase in the next decade as this group nears retirement age.

Strategies to address the faculty shortage are being sought nationwide among faculty in academic settings. These strategies include aggressive marketing within nursing and to the public, developing financial incentives and scholarships, including the support of federal funding such as the recently passed Nurse Reinvestment Act, and retaining senior faculty utilizing strategies similar to those being proposed for retaining the older nurse discussed in Chapter 7, "The Older Nurse." For a comprehensive discussion of the faculty shortage, including strategies to address it, read "Faculty Shortages Intensify Nation's Nursing Deficit" by logging on to *aacn.nche.edu/Publications/*.[2]

This is an opportune time for nurses interested in academic careers. Watch for recruitment incentives such as federally-funded master's and doctoral programs to be more available. To learn more about this read, "A Continuing Challenge: The Shortage of Educationally Prepared Nursing Faculty" in the *Online Journal of Nursing Issues* at *nursingworld.org/ojin/topic14/tpc14_3.htm*.[3]

WHAT TO WATCH FOR

Crises create opportunities not previously available, and the nursing shortage is no exception. The recruitment and education of nurses has become an urgently important priority for the nursing profession:

- Schools and colleges of nursing are amplifying their efforts to recruit eligible students by expanding their programs and increasing the flexibility of class schedules to meet the needs of busy students. Watch for innovative programs and the increased availability of distance-learning programs where you can take courses online.

- Special recruitment campaigns are being developed to recruit men and minority students, both of which are underrepresented populations in the nursing profession. You can track programs of interest though ANA (*nursingworld.org*), AACN (*aacn.nche.edu*), as well as the website of the journal *Minority Nurse* (*minoritynurse.com*). The Spring 2002 issue of this publication featured excellent articles on issues related to men and minorities.

- Take advantage of the increased availability of financial assistance and loan forgiveness programs. One example is the Nurse Reinvestment Act that was signed into law on August 1, 2002, by President Bush. The bill authorizes increased loans for nursing students and for nurses seeking advanced degrees. Two of the many nursing websites that will track the progress of this funding, including its availability, the dollar amount allotted, and the stipulations for eligibility are the American Nurses Association (*nursingworld.org*) and the American Association of Colleges of Nursing (*aacn.nche.edu*). You will find additional information about financial assistance in the Resources section.

- Watch for healthcare organizations to offer incentives for nursing education, especially for advanced practice roles that are anticipated to be in very short supply as the need for primary care increases.

LEVELS OF NURSING EDUCATION

The American Association of Colleges of Nursing (AACN) specifies three levels of education for the preparation of professional nurses. These are the baccalaureate, master's, and doctoral degrees. Although the baccalaureate is the primary pathway to professional nursing practice that is preferred among healthcare employers and offers the greatest career mobility for the nurse, there are two other entryways: the two-year associate's degree in nursing and the three-year hospital diploma, which has been steadily declining and currently represents only 10 percent of nursing educational programs at the basic level.[4] The educational preparation and subsequent roles and responsibilities these nurses have in nursing practice are described next. The back of this book provides resources for you to locate programs that will suit your needs and interests, including information on financing your nursing education.

The Baccalaureate and the Associate's Degree Nurse

Roles and Responsibilities

Upon graduation both of these nurses are considered entry-level practitioners, functioning as generalists and typically providing direct patient care. At this beginning level, they are both prepared to ensure coordinated and comprehensive care by collaborating closely with other healthcare personnel.

Educational Preparation: The B.S.N. vs the A.D.N.

There are issues related to educational entry into professional nursing practice that need to be understood if you are to assure yourself of the most thorough preparation and the greatest access to the options and opportunities in the healthcare marketplace.

There is a long-existing controversy within the nursing profession about which of the three educational pathways to becoming a professional nurse should be the standard. The debate has existed since at least 1965 when the American Nurses Association published a position paper stating that the B.S.N. should be the preferred entry mechanism and requirement for licensure. The position paper further stated that the graduate prepared at the baccalaureate level should be called a "professional nurse," while the associate's degree graduate be called a "technical nurse."

The debate about this issue within the profession has gone unresolved to this day, with advocates for each side holding strong to their beliefs. The fact that graduates from both programs are eligible for state licensure and have identical roles and responsibilities in nursing practice at the direct-care, generalist level (but not at the specialist level, in advanced practice, or in academic or management roles) only adds to the confusion for everyone, nurses, patients, and the larger healthcare community as well.

Features of the Bachelor's Degree in Nursing

The bachelor's degree program is typically four years in length and provides a liberal college education in the sciences and humanities along with preparation for nursing. The B.S.N. curriculum includes a strong focus on the development of intellectual skills, as well as scientific, critical thinking, humanistic, communication, and leadership skills. Courses in community health and research are also requirements in baccalaureate education that are omitted from the associate's degree program.

Following the first two years of liberal arts studies, students begin learning nursing theory, along with nursing skills and competencies in classes that combine theoretical and clinical components. While technical skills are essential to nursing practice, baccalaureate education emphasizes the additional importance of problem solving and establishes the basis for using clinical judgment.

Features of the Associate's Degree in Nursing

The associate's degree program is typically two years in length and offered at community colleges. While two years is devoted to the development of nursing skills and competencies as in the B.S.N. program, what is less emphasized and/or omitted entirely from the curriculum (in addition to research and community health) is the broader and deeper development of leadership, problem solving, and critical thinking skills. Hence, these nurses do well at providing direct patient care but are not well prepared for the leadership roles of charge nurse or team leader in the same way as the baccalaureate graduate is. Healthcare employers affirm this by requiring nurses who function at the case manager or supervisor level to be baccalaureate prepared. The A.D.N. graduate will also not be as qualified for employment in community nursing positions, such as home healthcare.

The A.D.N. program was originally developed to prepare "technical nurses" who had broader functions than the licensed practical nurse but a narrower scope of practice than the "professional nurse." The program evolved from the doctoral dissertation of Mildred Montag, Ed.D., R.N., a nurse educator.

Over the years the original intent and philosophy of the program has changed from being a terminal degree to developing "articulation" opportunities for these nurses to "complete" their education, as is the philosophical preference among the nursing leadership that supports baccalaureate education for entry into practice. These articulation programs are described later in this chapter.

The A.D.N. as an Entryway, not an End

The A.D.N. is a faster and less expensive entryway into professional nursing practice than the B.S.N. degree but has its limitations. It is a great starting point but you would be wise to carefully weigh the result of allowing this to remain your terminal degree, meaning the only formal preparation you have to offer a healthcare employer.

Be clear about the potential limitations of the associate's degree and commit yourself to adding the B.S.N. credential, either through the articulation programs described later in this chapter, or after working for a period of time as a direct care nurse and then returning to school. Nurses who choose this method of nursing education can often benefit from the tuition reimbursement offered by their employers if they return to school part time and continue working. See the following graph for a forecast of job openings for nurses with higher degrees.

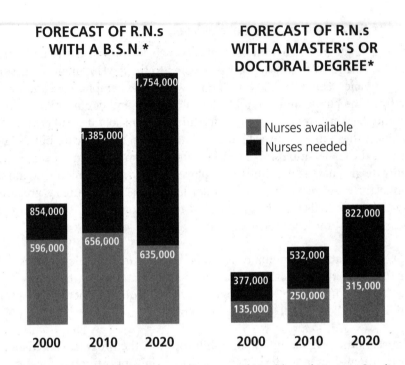

FORECAST OF R.N.s WITH A B.S.N.*

1,754,000
1,385,000
854,000
596,000
656,000
635,000

FORECAST OF R.N.s WITH A MASTER'S OR DOCTORAL DEGREE*

Nurses available
Nurses needed

822,000
532,000
377,000
315,000
250,000
135,000

2000   2010   2020   2000   2010   2020

*Bureau of Health Professions, U.S. Dept. of Health and Human Services

To understand this issue further, log on to *aacn.nche.edu*, the website of the American Association of Colleges of Nursing and read "Your Nursing Career: A Look At The Facts." A paragraph from that publication appears below, summarizing the findings of the National Advisory Council on Nurse Education and Practice. Combine this statement with the information about employment opportunities along the "continuum of care" which you will find in Chapter 11, "The Market Research Department of *You, Inc.*" This will arm you with the information you need to make informed decisions about your nursing education.

> "Baccalaureate nursing programs are far more likely than other entry level tracks to provide students with onsite clinical training in noninstitutional settings outside the hospital. As a result, the B.S.N. graduate is well prepared for practice in such sites as home health agencies, outpatient centers, and neighborhood clinics where opportunities are expanding as hospitals focus more on acute care, and health services move beyond the hospital to more primary and preventive care throughout the community."

Further validation comes from the Bureau of Labor Statistics (*bls.gov*) in the 2002–2003 edition of their Occupational Outlook Handbook:

> "Individuals considering nursing school should weigh carefully the pros and cons of enrolling in a B.S.N. program because, if they do so, their advancement opportunities usually are broader. In fact, some career paths are open only to nurses with bachelor's or advanced degrees. A bachelor's degree is often necessary for administrative positions, and it is a prerequisite for admission to graduate nursing programs in research, consulting, teaching, or a clinical specialization."

The Master's-Prepared Nurse

Roles and Responsibilities

The nurse who desires clinical, academic, or administrative advancement will need a master's degree and possibly a doctoral degree as well. Admission to graduate nursing programs requires a baccalaureate degree. The master's-prepared nurse functions in advanced practice roles, including health promotion, the management and delivery of primary healthcare, and case management of the acutely or chronically ill patient. This nurse is also prepared for roles in community health and administration.

Nurses prepared at the master's level are qualified to become managers and administrators of healthcare organizations, including the directors of divisions and departments of nursing and nursing services. Increasingly, the doctoral degree is preferred for administrators and nurse executives, along with the Master of Business Administration (M.B.A.). Many nurse administrators/executives add the M.B.A. to their master's and doctoral preparation in nursing.

Master's-prepared nurses are also qualified to teach in colleges and schools of nursing, although are often limited to adjunct faculty roles, including the education and supervision of nursing students during their clinical rotations. For nurses seeking full-time, tenure-track academic appointments, the doctoral degree will be necessary.

The master's degree also prepares the advanced practice nurse who can function in the following roles:

Nurse Practitioner (N.P.)

These nurses provide all primary care services, including administration of immunization protocols, ordering and interpreting x-rays and laboratory data, and so on. They practice in a variety of specialties such as adult health, pediatrics, women's health, family health, as well as psychiatry and mental health. They can prescribe medications in all states, with 18 states authorizing this practice as an independent function without requiring physician collaboration. They work in clinics and hospitals in metropolitan and rural areas, especially in places with underserved healthcare needs, and in private practice as well. Professional certification is usually required by employers and insurance companies that provide reimbursement of healthcare expenses. The N.P. has more broadly defined functions when compared to the C.N.S. (see below).

Clinical Nurse Specialist (C.N.S.)

This nurse has highly specialized skills and is prepared to practice in a wide variety of nursing areas including psychiatric/mental health, community health, oncology, pediatrics, and so on. Primary roles in which the C.N.S. functions often include acting as a patient advocate, as well as educator, clinical resource, consultant and role model to other nurses, especially those practicing at the generalist level. C.N.S.s can be found in all employment sectors of the healthcare industry as well as in private practice; the psychiatric clinical nurse specialist often has his or her own practice. Like the N.P., professional certification is typically required or advantageous.

Certified Nurse Midwife (C.N.M.)

This nurse graduates from an accredited nurse midwifery program and provides prenatal care, labor and delivery care, neonatal care, family planning, and well-woman care. The C.N.M. has a formal, collaborative relationship with an obstetrician who provides consultation as well as management of high-risk patients. C.N.M.s are employed in hospitals, freestanding clinics and birth centers, ambulatory sites, and physician's offices. Professional certification is required.

Certified Registered Nurse Anesthetist (C.R.N.A.)

This master's-prepared nurse graduates from a certified nurse anesthesia program and administers anesthetic agents, provides pre- and postanesthesia care, performs emergency resuscitation, and acute and chronic pain management. Employment settings include hospitals, surgicenters, emergency rooms, and physician's offices. Professional certification is required.

Educational Preparation

The typical master's degrees granted include:

- M.S., Master of Science with a nursing major, such as psychiatric/mental health
- M.S.N., Master of Science in Nursing
- M.N.Sc., Master in Nursing Science
- M.Ed., Master in Education with a major in nursing, such as teaching/learning
- M.A., Master of Arts with a major in nursing, such as administration
- M.P.H., Master of Public Health with a nursing major, such as community health

The Nurse Prepared at the Doctoral Level

Roles and Responsibilities

Doctoral programs prepare nurses to expand and contribute to the nursing knowledge base through scholarly work, research, advanced practice, nursing/healthcare administration, and/or teaching. A doctoral-prepared nurse is an influential leader who can have roles in a variety of healthcare and academic settings, for example, as a nurse executive leading the nursing division and its related healthcare services in a major medical center or as the dean and/or tenured professor in a university-based college of nursing program.

Educational Preparation

The doctoral degrees that are typically granted include:

- Ph.D., Doctor of Philosophy
- Ed.D., Doctor of Education
- D.N.Sc., or D.N.S., Doctor of Nursing Science

SOLUTIONS TO BARRIERS TO NURSING EDUCATION

While many practicing nurses and students desire the B.S.N. if they don't already have it, they typically cite the following barriers:

- The cost of tuition
- Time factors, especially the ability to match the time they have available with the hours classes are offered
- Confusion or lack of knowledge about program options and requirements
- Already in possession of a baccalaureate degree in another field

Educational institutions and healthcare organizations are taking steps to reduce these barriers, especially in light of their commitment to facilitate student recruitment as a strategy to address the nursing shortage. The programs that are described below provide solutions to these and other barriers that make nursing education in the 21st century increasingly accessible, especially as the influence of computers and the Internet finds its way deeper and deeper into our professional lives.

Articulation Programs

These are sometimes called "degree-completion" programs, in which a signed agreement between a baccalaureate program and an associate degree program provide a kind of seamless pipeline for the A.D.N. graduate to obtain the B.S.N. degree.

The collaborative efforts of and agreements between a particular A.D.N. and B.S.N. program permit the advancement of the A.D.N. student's education in the most facilitative way possible. Because of the predetermined collaborative efforts of both educational institutions, students are ensured the best use of both programs. The result is a win-win outcome for the student as well as for the educational programs, in that time and money are utilized most efficiently and credits are not needlessly lost.

Articulation agreements can vary greatly. To take advantage of this important educational option, it will be necessary to inquire about it from the A.D.N. and/or B.S.N. programs in which you are interested.

Another version of the articulation program, sometimes called "three plus one," allows the A.D.N. graduate to complete the liberal arts requirements at their community college by staying on for a third year, transfering these credits to a B.S.N. program to which they have been accepted, and then completing the B.S.N. requirements in the fourth year.

Accelerated B.S.N. Programs

For students who have a baccalaureate degree in another field, this accelerated B.S.N. option could be an excellent choice, particularly for people interested in nursing as a second career. Typically, students attend classes full time from 8 AM to 4 PM, five days per week and earn a B.S.N. in 13 months, although programs vary in length between 12 and 18 months. The curriculum contains the same courses and clinical hour requirements as the traditional B.S.N. program, but is more compact, and as a result more rigorous, as well as intellectually and physically demanding.

You will find additional information about these programs, including a comprehensive list of accelerated baccalaureate programs in the AACN *Issue Bulletin* entitled "Accelerated Programs: The Fast-Track to Careers in Nursing" at *aacn.nche.edu/ Publications/issues/Aug02.htm.*

Generic Master's Programs

This is a program for people who are not yet nurses, have completed a degree at the baccalaureate or graduate level in another field, and have decided on a career in a clinical, administrative, or academic advanced practice role that they are already aware requires master's level preparation. These are people who are clear about their nursing career goals, have investigated their options carefully, and are looking for the most facilitative path to achieve them.

The program composition varies from school to school; some may be completed in four semesters, including one semester that requires a five-day per week, three-month-long clinical internship. Like the accelerated B.S.N. programs, students enrolling in these programs need to be prepared for an intellectually and physically demanding educational challenge.

For additional information about these programs, including a comprehensive list of accelerated master's programs, see the AACN *Issue Bulletin* entitled "Accelerated Programs: The Fast-Track to Careers in Nursing" at *aacn.nche.edu/ Publications/issues/Aug02.htm.*

DISTANCE LEARNING PROGRAMS

As familiarity with the computer and the Internet increase, and high-speed communication links among people become more commonplace and indispensable, traditional face-to-face education is being supplemented, or in some cases, replaced with online learning in virtual rather than "brick and mortar" classrooms. Students, including those in nursing programs, increasingly have the option of online as well as traditional education courses and programs. Online education, distance learning, and distance education are the terms used to describe the learning that occurs in classrooms that are virtual rather than real.

In their online publication called "Distance Education: A Consumer's Guide," the Western Cooperative for Educational Telecommunications (WCET) defines distance education as:

> "Instruction that occurs when the instructor and student are separated by distance or time, or both. A wide array of technologies is currently being used to link the instructor and student. Courses are offered via videotape, broadcast television, ITFS (Instructional Television Fixed Service), microwave, satellite, interactive video, audio tapes, audio-conferencing, CD-ROM, and increasingly, networking—including email, the Internet, and its World Wide Web."

This guide is a very helpful resource for those contemplating online education and can be accessed at: (*wcet.info/resources/publications/conguide/conguida.htm*). The following topics are covered in the guide, the exploration of which will allow for a thorough assessment of your readiness for this type of learning, including how to get started:

- Who are distance learners?
- Where do I begin?
- How do I choose a school?
- How do I evaluate quality?
- What is accreditation?
- Even if a school is accredited, how do I make sure its electronically offered programs are of high quality?
- How do I evaluate a program from a school that is not accredited?
- What is the best technology to use?
- Making a decision

- For more information: some published guides
- Resources on the Internet
- Higher education regional accrediting bodies

According to WCET's guide, students who enroll in distance learning courses require the skills and attributes listed below. Place a check mark next to the ones you believe you have:

❏ Good time management skills

❏ Self-motivation and discipline

❏ Comfort with using a computer

❏ Flexible learning styles

❏ Motivation

Distance learning courses are highly interactive experiences with direct access to teachers and classmates through email communication. They contain the same objectives, workload, assignments, and expectations as classroom options except that the student can choose the time of day and for how long he or she will attend the "virtual" class to fulfill the requirements. The clinical practice component, if required, is taught close to the student's home by qualified nurse preceptors at local healthcare organizations that are chosen carefully and evaluated by the degree-granting institution. This kind of choice and control in relation to time management makes distance education an extremely attractive option for busy 21st-century nurses.

Additional features and benefits of distance learning are described in the introductory materials of the websites of online universities. For example, at the Duquesne University home page (*nursing.duq.edu*) you can read about these important features of online education:

> "Studies show that learning at a distance can increase the student's retention by lowering social barriers and engaging the student more so than in a physical setting. The use of the written word, through email, as a means of communication forces the student to put coherent thoughts together and reflect on the course material. Because email communication is instantaneous and easy to apply, the student has direct communication with the professor—something that is not always possible in the classroom."

To have an actual experience of online learning, The University of Colorado Health Sciences Center, School of Nursing (*www2.uchsc.edu/*) invites you to "test-drive" a sample R.N. to B.S. course, called "ROOTS," an acronym for "Reach Out Online to Succeed." Once you arrive at the home page of this course, you can interact with the features all online courses have in common, including the syllabus and a course module, audio features, bulletin board discussions, and online quizzes. The course also provides an excellent interactive, 20 question, multiple-choice quiz to test your readiness for learning online. A sample question is:

> The type of learning environment that I learn best in is:
>
> ❏ An independent study environment offering self-taught learning
>
> ❏ A student-centered environment: I'm on my own but have help as needed
>
> ❏ A teacher-directed environment with all materials explained in detail

In Chapter 4, "The Nurse and Technology," you will find another online nursing course to explore called "Nursing and the Internet." Additional resources will be found at the back of this book.

Examples of Online Nursing Education

There are ever-increasing numbers and varieties of online educational options, including degree programs, continuing education programs, and certificate programs. Nearly every nursing degree program offers courses or its complete program online and is accredited by AACN (American Association of Colleges in Nursing) and NLN (National League for Nursing).

Some examples of degree and certificate programs and what they offer are:

> **Duquesne University** (*nursing.duq.edu*)
> R.N. to B.S.N./M.S.N.
> Post-B.S.N. Certificates
> M.S.N.
> Post-Master's Certificates
> Ph.D.

> **Drexel University e-Learning** (*drexel.com*)
> R.N. to B.S.N.
> R.N. to B.S.N. to M.S.N.
> M.S.N. in Nursing Education
> M.S.N. in Public Health

M.S.N. in Leadership and Management
M.S.N. in Clinical Trials
M.S.N. completion for Nurse Practitioners
Certificate in Education
Certificate in Leadership and Management
Certificate in Clinical Trials
Registered Nurse First Assistant Program

Jacksonville University (*jacksonvilleu.com*)
R.N. to B.S.N., entirely online

Kaplan University (*kaplan.com*)
R.N. to B.S.N.

University of Phoenix Online (*phoenix.edu*)
B.S. in Healthcare Services
B.S.N.
M.B.A. in Healthcare Management
M.S. in Nursing
M.S. in Nursing/M.B.A. in Healthcare Management

CONTINUING EDUCATION

The educational preparation of degree-granting programs (B.S.N., master's, etc.) arms the nurse with basic information and provides him or her with a foundation upon which to build a nursing practice. Ongoing continuing education (CE) ensures that this information stays current so that nursing skills and competencies are effectively and safely employed.

A life-long commitment to professional education is not only a hallmark of the professional nurse, but extremely important in light of rapidly changing and emerging technologies, as well as the explosion of discoveries in health and science. It also ensures that that mindset and attitude of the nurse changes and develops over time, an essential characteristic for nurses who seek to influence others and utilize relatedness in their work.

While continuing education is the nurse's professional and ethical responsibility, it is also frequently mandated for license renewal by the boards of nursing of each state. Since these CE requirements differ greatly from state to state, each nurse must keep track of the current and sometimes changing requirements. Each of the state nurses' associations or the state boards of nursing will provide this information on their websites or in writing as requested. For a listing of the state boards of nursing, including their websites, refer to the back of this book. An additional way to determine what your requirements might be is through one of the nursing-specific sites that provide career information such as *Nursing Spectrum* (*nursingspectrum.com*). Some examples of state CE requirements are:

Alabama: 24 contact hours every renewal period

Hawaii: CE not required

Texas: 20 contact hours every two years

Utah: One of the following every two years required for license renewal: 30 contact hours or 200 practice hours; or, 15 contact hours or 400 practice hours.

For nurses that are board certified by ANCC (American Nurses Credentialing Center) or by nursing specialty associations, continuing education along with a specified number of practice hours is mandatory for recertification. This information can be obtained at ANCC's website: *nursecredentialing.org*, and at the websites of the specialty associations by which you are certified.

Some organizations that offer continuing education programs are:

Nursing Center (*nursingcenter.com*)
Select your own CE topic using the site's search engine. Offerings include:
- Outcomes Research: An Interdisciplinary Perspective
- Right Ventricular Myocardial Infarction: When Power Fails
- Diversity Issues in the Delivery of Healthcare

New York State Nurses Association (*nysna.org*)
Offerings include:
- Preventing Medication Errors
- End of Life Care
- Domestic Violence: The Nurse's Role

SUNY Stony Brook School of Nursing (*nursing.stonybrook.edu*)
Select CE topic of interest using their search engine. Offerings include:

- Cost Analysis in the Healthcare Arena
- Infant Security in the Maternal and Pediatric Settings
- Helping Nurses Publish in Nursing Journals

Nursing Spectrum (*nursingspectrum.com*)
Offerings include:

- Abdominal Aortic Aneurysm
- Earning Degrees by Distance Education
- Psychiatric Nursing in Correctional Settings

RnCeus.com (*rnceus.com*)
Offerings include:

- Hormones in Pregnancy
- Understanding Coagulation Tests
- Biochemical Terrorism: An Emergency Room Resource

To explore many more of these options, type in "online nursing education" at any search engine (refer to Chapter 4, "The Nurse and Technology," for more about how to do this). Search engines that are nursing-specific will provide you with many lists of CE programs. Nursing-specific search engines can be found at: *UltimateNurse.com, Nursing.advanceweb.com/main.aspx, NursingSpectrum.com,* and *nursingworld.org.*

THE NCLEX-R.N.® EXAM

NCLEX-RN® stands for National Council Licensure Examination for Registered Nurses. This exam is required to obtain a license to practice as an R.N. You may have heard people use the term "state boards" when referring to this exam. This is really a misnomer. The R.N. licensure exam, or NCLEX-RN® exam, is a nationally standardized exam that is given in all parts of the United States. The purpose of the exam is to *safeguard the public*. It determines if you are a safe and effective nurse. It tests for minimum competency to practice nursing.

The test content is based on the knowledge and activities of an entry-level nurse. The test questions are written by nursing faculty and clinical specialists and are based on integrated nursing content—not on the medical model of medical, surgical, obstetrics, pediatrics, and psychiatric nursing. This is different from the way courses are organized at most nursing programs where there are separate medical, surgical, pediatric, psychiatric, and obstetric classes. The NCLEX-RN® exam asks integrated questions because in the "real world," patients have multiple problems and needs.

What information will be tested on the NCLEX-RN® exam? The exam is based on entry-level practice, not high-tech or advanced nursing care. For example, Swans Gantz catheters are considered high-tech nursing care and questions about them are usually not found on the exam. Questions involving the transfer of a patient with right-sided weakness from the bed to the chair is knowledge that is necessary for a nurse to know to be safe and effective. Questions concerning this topic may appear on the exam.

The CAT (Computer Adaptive Test) adapts to your knowledge, skills, and ability level. The computer selects questions based on the difficulty level of the question and the area of the test plan. Think of it as a line drawn in your computer. This is the level of knowledge a nurse needs to know to be safe and effective. As you go above the line, questions get harder and require more than just minimum competency knowledge. As you go below the line, the questions get easier and require less than minimum competency knowledge. The farther you go above the line, the harder the questions get. The lower you go below the line, the easier the questions get. The line that is minimum competency was recently raised. That means the exam is harder to pass now. You need to correctly answer more difficult questions to pass the NCLEX-RN® exam. Good preparation for this high-stakes exam is essential.

The question sequence is determined interactively. The computer selects what is considered to be a relatively easy first question. The next question is selected by the computer based the accuracy on your response. If your answer is correct, the next question is slightly more difficult. If your answer is wrong, the next question is slightly easier.

You will answer a minimum of 75 questions to a maximum of 265 questions. Your exam will end when one of three things happens: 1) When the computer has determined your ability level, or 2) When you have completed a maximum of six hours of testing time, or 3) When you have answered a maximum of 265 questions.

The exam is pass/fail. No numbers are generated by the system. The NCLEX-RN® exam is a test of minimum competency to practice nursing, not a nursing achievement test. There is not a certain percentage of the questions that you need to get right. The people who write the exam say that at the end of the exam, everyone is getting about half of the questions correct—that's 50 percent. The difference is that the people who pass the exam are getting half of the harder questions correct, and the people who fail the exam are getting half of the easier questions correct. When you start getting one right, then one wrong because they have increased the level of difficulty, then one right, and then one wrong, your exam will end because the computer has figured out the level of difficulty of questions you are able to consistently answer correctly.

There is no penalty for guessing on this exam. If you don't know the answer, try eliminating some of the answer choices and then guess! You must answer a question before the next question will appear on the computer screen.

Everyone who takes the NCLEX-RN® exam will see 15 experimental questions. These questions are not counted, but are being tested for future exams. You can't tell which questions are experimental, so do your best on each and every question.

You will schedule a date and time to take the NCLEX-RN® exam at a NCS Pearson Testing Center, and will complete the exam in one day at one sitting. The results of the NCLEX-RN® exam will not be made available to you at the exam site, but will be sent to you in about two to four weeks from your State Board of Nursing.

Most of you are familiar with nursing school questions written at the recall and recognition level of ability. With these questions, you read the question stem, recall or remember the answer, go to the answer choices looking for a particular answer, and recognize the correct answer. Most questions on the NCLEX-RN® exam are written at the application and analysis level of difficulty. This means that when you read the question, you are unsure of what the question is asking. For some questions you know what the question is asking, but you don't recognize the correct answer choice. To correctly answer questions at the application and analysis level of difficulty, you need to use critical thinking skills.

A sample test question appears below, taken from Kaplan's *NCLEX-RN® Exam*:

Question:

Which of the following actions, if performed by the nurse, would be considered negligence?

(1)   Obtaining a Guthrie blood test on a 4-day-old infant.
(2)   Massaging lotion on the abdomen of a 3-year-old diagnosed with Wilm's tumor.
(3)   Instructing a 5-year-old asthmatic to blow on a pinwheel.
(4)   Playing kickball with a 10-year-old with juvenile arthritis (JA).

Explanation:

REWORDED QUESTION: What is an incorrect behavior?

STRATEGY: Think about the consequence of each action.

NEEDED INFO: Negligence is the unintentional failure of a nurse to perform an act that a reasonable person would or would not perform in similar circumstances; can be an act of commission or omission. Standards of care: the actions that other nurses would do in the same or similar circumstances that provide for quality client care. Nurse practice acts: state laws that determine the scope of the practice of nursing.

CATEGORY: Analysis/Safe and Effective Care

(1) Obtaining a Guthrie blood test on a 4-day-old infant—*obtain after ingestion of protein, no later than 7 days after delivery*

(2) Massaging lotion on the abdomen of a 3-year-old diagnosed with Wilm's tumor—**CORRECT: manipulation of mass may cause dissemination of cancer cells**

(3) Instructing a 5-year-old asthmatic to blow on a pinwheel—*exercise that will extend expiratory time and increase expiratory pressure*

(4) Playing kickball with a 10-year-old with juvenile arthritis (JA)—*excellent moving and stretching exercise*

Now that you're knowledgeable about the NCLEX-RN® exam, let's talk about how to prepare for this exam. Preparation for the NCLEX-RN® exam entails a systematic review of nursing content, and application of nursing care principles. Because the exam covers all areas in nursing with emphasis on safe care and minimum competency, you should review the entire nursing curriculum to prepare for the exam. Most nursing students take a review course, and buy a book or software program. Review courses are helpful because they provide a structured time for study, and ensure that all necessary content is reviewed. The largest provider of NCLEX-RN® exam preparation is Kaplan (*kaplannursing.com*) which provides online and classroom courses along with preparation materials such as a question bank and Kaplan's *NCLEX-RN® Exam* book that contains a computer-based practice test in addition to over a hundred additional practice questions.

Additional information about the NCLEX-RN® exam can be found at *kaplannursing.com*, including:

- Taking the CAT
- Learn Client Needs
- Your Results
- How to Register
- Alternate Question Types

CONTINUING THE JOURNEY

Lucille Joel, R.N., Ed.D., F.A.A.N., a renowned nursing leader and educator, believes a long-standing problem in the nursing profession that erodes the professional image of the registered nurse is that "nurses have traditionally derived their identity from their statutory title, R.N., rather than from their academic preparation."[5] Committing yourself to lifelong nursing education in all its variations will go a long way in returning the individual and collective professional nursing identity to within the nurse where it belongs rather than on the piece of paper, the license, that represents it.

CHAPTER 4

The Nurse and Technology

What do you think about the presence of technology in your personal and professional life as the years of the 21st century unfold, and with it, the promise of more and more technological wonders? Do you see technology as:

❏ invasive	or	❏ supportive?
❏ threatening	or	❏ challenging?
❏ friend	or	❏ foe?

Whatever you think about technology and its ubiquity in your life, it is here to stay. None of us get to decide *whether* we will have a relationship with technology, only the *kind* of relationship it will be. *In your nursing practice, you may be able to choose low-tech vs. high-tech work, but there is no longer any such thing as "no-tech."*

Before reading further, take the following quiz to determine what kind of relationship you currently have with technology.

How many of these technological experiences are in your life?

Professional Life

❏ Computers for documentation
❏ PDAs with drug information
❏ EKG readings over the telephone
❏ Computerized staff schedules

Personal Life

❏ Cell phones
❏ Beepers and pagers
❏ Computers and the Internet
❏ Television and radio

❏ Hand-held heart rate doppler

❏ Hand-held ultrasound for bedside bladder assessment

List others:

❏ _____

❏ VCRs and DVDs

❏ Video cameras

List others:

❏ _____

How many of these technological advances, just over the horizon in healthcare, do you know about or are already working with?

❏ Robotic surgery

❏ Artificial blood

❏ Electronic bra to diagnose breast cancer

❏ Transcranial magnetic stimulation to treat depression

❏ Genome advances

❏ Brain pacemakers to treat Parkinson's disease

❏ Vest to record and diagnose cardiac and respiratory disease

Identify three things you love about technology:

_____

_____

_____

Identify three things you hate about technology:

_____

_____

_____

Check the box next to the statement below that most closely identifies your relationship with technology:

- ❏ I love it. I can't get enough of it. I find it easy. I'm the first one among my friends to buy the latest update or newest technological marvel. At work, peers and colleagues often turn to me for assistance with technology.

- ❏ I've made my peace with technology since I can't escape it, but I wish the "next new thing" would wait until I finish learning how to use the last "next new thing," which works perfectly well anyway.

- ❏ I don't go near it unless I have to. I think it's the scourge of society, ruining the imaginative lives of our children and filling our landfills with unnecessary and nonbiodegradable waste that is a legacy of which we should be ashamed. I'm proud of the fact and don't mind telling you that I don't own a computer and never will!

If you responded by checking the last statement above and you want to work as a nurse in the 21st century, you're in trouble. Your challenge will be to convince everyone around you to see your point of view, or decide to ride the horse in the direction it's going, forward, that is, farther and farther into technological territories.

You're in good company, however, if your responses to these statements combined elements of all three of them, representing the kind of love-hate relationship with technology that a majority of people have, aware that as it simplifies their lives, so does it make them more complex. Our relationship with technology may best be described as a bit Dickensian: it provides us with the "best of times and the worst of times."

In this chapter you will find information about the influence and presence of technology in your nursing practice, as well as how to utilize the Internet for managing your career. This will assist you in strengthening your relationship to the technology you can no longer avoid and determine ways to use it to your advantage. You will find additional discussions about the stress, sensory overload, and over-connectedness that accompany our relationships with technology in Chapter 16, "The Resilient Nurse: Self-Care Strategies."

THE 20th CENTURY: THE VERY RECENT PAST

Twentieth-century nurses, many of whom are still practicing today, were witness to the technological explosion in the healthcare workplace. The technology "invasion" started in a small way with digital thermometers that replaced the glass-mercury ones and then IV pumps that electronically monitored infusion rates, soon skyrocketing into more and more complicated and sophisticated monitoring and life-support machinery.

As the march of technology proceeded, it was soon evident that specialized care and monitoring would be needed for patients who were becoming more and more tethered to invasive, computerized, and centrally located "lines." The intensive care units were born and many nurses began specializing in combining their familiar high-touch skills with their new high-tech ones.

Technology changed procedures like cardiac catheterization. Sonograms allowed a much improved peek into interior body spaces. CT scans and PET scans revealed even more information, allowing faster and more precise diagnoses and treatment. Laser surgery was born, and laporoscopic surgery began replacing traditional surgery allowing patients to go home sooner and less sick.

This may sound like ancient history to the younger generations of nurses whose familiarity with technology is like breathing, but the 25 years or so that it has taken for technology to transform healthcare is hardly long enough to qualify as ancient.

THE 21st CENTURY: THE PRESENT HURTLING INTO THE FUTURE

Fast-forward to the 21st century and what once seemed dazzling pales in comparison to now. The most important technological skill the 21st-century nurse needs has less to do with learning how to work the latest technological marvel and more to do with adapting quickly to the obsolescence of it, always ready for the inevitable "what's new and what's next."

The 21st-century nurse is technologically proficient, computer literate, and Internet savvy. This nurse may not know how to manage every piece of technology he or she comes across but is ready, willing, and able to master it quickly, without thinking twice about it.

To get a glimpse into how technology has infiltrated and influenced 21st-century nursing practice, follow Ida and Sam, two medical-surgical nurses, for part of their workday. How close are their activities to yours? Or, to how you would like to be working as a nurse?

Two 21st-Century Nurses: Ida and Sam

Ida and Sam use the hospital's computer-based Intranet system, the internal Internet, to communicate with and send information to the hospital's various departments. A physician's order is immediately printed out as a request in the radiology department, pharmacy, or laboratory, allowing Sam and Ida more time to focus on patient care issues. Bar-coded information is returned with the lab results, reducing the chance of error.

During his orientation, Sam was amused to find the old pneumatic tube system intact and still used to send laboratory and pharmacy requests when the computer terminal goes down, which thankfully is happening less often now that the system was finally upgraded. Ida is among the older generation of nurses, straddling the worlds of the 20th and 21st centuries, who takes some gleeful satisfaction when this happens, teasing Sam about what she thinks is his overconnectedness to and overreliance upon technology. Despite their teasing, they are great allies and resources to one another. Sam has helped Ida with the technology that sometimes baffles her, while Ida has mentored Sam, only a two-year veteran of nursing, and watched him grow more comfortable in his role.

Ida uses the computer at the bedside and/or the nursing station for patient documentation and to obtain prior medical records, often marveling at how quickly she can access information that once took so much more time. Gone are the forms to fill out and the calls to make to request medical records. While not foolproof nor available for as much information as she'd like, quite a lot of the patient information is readily inputted and updated using the hospital's sophisticated data entry program. Her friend Barbara is a psychiatric home care nurse and uses a laptop with drop-down menus to check off appropriate words related to the patient's status rather than writing long paragraphs. Barbara also uses specialized software to schedule patients for office and clinic visits, treatments, and surgery, bragging about how much time she saves by doing it this way.

Sam told Ida about the continuing education program he recently attended regarding the hospital's new policy on privacy and confidentiality of computerized medical records. The hospital will be implementing the privacy standards mandated by the new Health Insurance Portability and Accountability Act. She will be attending the class next week but her interest was piqued and she intends to read about this when she's online over the weekend on the Internet site Sam received from the class and gave her (*cms.hhs.gov/hipaa/*).

Sam has been teaching a newly diagnosed diabetic patient how to give himself insulin injections and is pleased to see how much the patient learned from the three online diabetic education sites he encouraged the patient to explore. This patient is a real Internet enthusiast and told Sam about many other sites that he found, some of which had different information than Sam gave him. Sam used this opportunity to caution the patient about carefully critiquing the many sites he'll find when surfing the Web, especially if he is reading a research study. He told the patient to use the following questions to determine the accuracy of the data: How current is the information? What are the credentials of the person or organization offering the information? How large was the research study and were the results duplicated anywhere? He gave the patient the following healthcare websites that could be trusted to provide accurate and up-to-date information:

- Mayo Clinic   *mayoclinic.com*
- U.S. Department of Health and   *healthfinder.gov*
  Human Services, Office of Disease
  Prevention and Health Promotion
- The American Heart Association   *americanheart.org*
- The National Institute of Health   *nih.gov*
- The American Diabetic Association   *diabetes.org*

Sam also showed this patient how to use email to contact a list of health providers specializing in diabetes that have home pages filled with good information and who would respond to email questions. Sam was pleased to hear that the patient's health insurance company had already registered him for their health-oriented email services.

Sam and Ida both use the hospital's access to the Internet for the reference tools and research-oriented websites they have come to rely on, especially when pressed for time and needing a fast answer to a clinical issue. Ida has finally stopped thumbing through her old, reliable print versions of what she can now find faster and more up-to-date online. Although she remembers her initial reticence to learn the computer five years ago, she can't imagine ever getting along without it now, at work or at home. Some of Sam and Ida's favorite reference tools are listed below. Sam accesses some of these sites using his PDA (personal digital assistant). Ida is holding out from developing a relationship with yet one more piece of technology, although the games she sees Sam play and the city maps he can access on it are looking more and more appealing to her.

Sam and Ida's Clinical Reference Tools

- Lippincott's Nursing Center   *nursingcenter.com/home/index.asp*
- *Online Journal of Issues in Nursing*   *nursingworld.org/ojin*
- Auscultation Assistant (hear actual   *wilkes.med.ucla.edu/intro.html* heart and breath sounds!!)
- Medlineplus   *medlineplus.gov*
- Nurses' PDR Resource List   *nursespdr.com*
- RxList   *rxlist.com*
- Nursing Care Plans   *nursingcareplans.com*
- Brownson's Nursing Notes   *members.tripod.com/~DianneBrownson*

Sam and Ida are each on different committees related to the hospital's technology initiatives. Sam is working with the hospital's IT (Information Technology) Department to set up a staff scheduling pattern that will work better for the needs of their unit than the centralized one they have been using.

Ida is one of the nursing representatives on the hospital's Telehealth Consortium that is part of the city-wide delivery of health information and services through the coordination of information, technology, and communication networks. Ida is thrilled to be able to use her long-standing interest and experience in patient education in this new way where it is possible to reach more people faster and easier with important health information, often without requiring a visit to a health provider. She will be an adviser to the hospital's new program in which their home care nurses will be using a hand-held computer with a camera to transmit patient care data to physicians at a distant site. Her friend Karen who works in the cardiac catheterization lab often tells her about the cardiac procedures that are video-conferenced to other counties for consultation as well as for medical education. She has begun to learn more about telehealth on various Internet sites, including the Office of Advancement of Telehealth (*telehealth.hrsa.gov*) that is committed to the development and investigation of the best ways to provide patients with electronic information technologies. She read the stories of many dramatic consultations using telemedicine at this site. The one that really excited her was the telemedicine consultation requested by a Family Nurse Practitioner:

From the Northern California Telemedicine Network (NCTN), Santa Rosa Memorial Hospital (SRMH), Santa Rosa, CA:

Case 1—Emergency Medicine

"This spring, a patient with a 5-6 cm laceration and crash injury to the forearm and hand was seen by a Family Nurse Practitioner (FNP) in a clinic in Gualala, CA. The patient worked at the local lumber mill and had caught his hand and forearm in the chain that moved wood through the mill. The FNP assessed the laceration and injury, and determined that the patient had a possible fracture and compartment syndrome. The FNP contacted SRMH Emergency Department (ED) for a telemedicine consult with an ED physician and radiologist.

Based on images that were transmitted with the general exam camera, it was determined that the patient did not need to be transported and the FNP would be able to clean, suture, and splint the wound on-site. The patient was saved a 5-hour roundtrip transport to SRMH and the expense of an ED visit. The patient, FNP, ED physician and radiologist rated the telemedicine consult as good (highest possible ranking). The FNP stated that the help from the radiologist was 'quick' and the service from the ED physician was 'excellent.'"

Recently, Ida and Sam shared their career goals with one another. Sam was investigating graduate nursing programs that prepared informatics nurses. He felt sure that combining his interest in and knack for technology with his growing nursing competency would make for a very satisfying career option. Ida was so inspired about the Family Nurse Practitioner's use of telehealth that she was once again considering becoming an advance practice nurse, as she had thought to do earlier in her career. She still wasn't sure this was the right move for her but what she found so interesting was that the thoughts of retiring that had preoccupied her these last few years had been replaced by ideas that would continue to expand her career rather than shut it down. Her interest in nursing had become reinvigorated by what she sees around her every day and what she knows is just around the corner. Why would she choose to miss any of it?

THE INTERNET: THE OTHER HEALTHCARE REVOLUTION

The age of information begun in the latter 20th century has broadened its impact in this new millennium in ways that could only be called revolutionary. Accessing and using information, the currency of these times, and staying connected to others through high-speed communication devices has forever changed the way we live and work. Those among you that find this revolting rather than revolutionary may be lost in a time warp that will marginalize your experiences and limit your involvement as the 21st century marches on.

Before reading further, review the list of commonly used Internet terms below and determine if you understand what they mean. This is not meant to be an all-inclusive list but rather some of the minimum information required to ensure that you can access Internet information and find your way around Internet territories. Use the information in this section to supplement what you already know or as an enticement to learn more. The definitions below were adapted from Webopedia, an online encyclopedia of computer and Internet terms *(webopedia.com).*

❏ Internet   A vast array of separate networks, maintained by individuals or organizations that are linked together, acting as a kind of unified whole for the purpose of sharing, transferring, transmitting, and communicating news, information, and services.

❏ World Wide Web   Abbreviated as "www," it is the system that provides access to information and services on the Internet, especially those offering multimedia and interactive properties.

❏ Search Engine   A program that searches documents for specific keywords and returns a list of these documents to the requester.

     ❏ Google   An example of a search engine

     ❏ Yahoo   An example of a search engine

     ❏ Excite   An example of a search engine

     ❏ Dogpile   An example of a search engine

❏ Bookmark   This means to mark a document or a specific place in a document for later retrieval; allows you to easily revisit this page at another time; a kind of landmark so that you don't get too lost (although getting lost can be half the fun, quite an adventure, and perhaps the best way to learn what the Internet is all about!).

❒ Listserv	An automatic mailing list server. Email is addressed to a listserv mailing list and then broadcast to everyone who subscribes to the list. This results in a newsgroup or forum, a kind of online community of people with particular interests.
❒ Email	Short for *electronic mail*, it is the transmission of messages over communication networks, the Internet.
❒ Modem	Short for *modulator-demodulator*, and means a device used by the computer to transmit data over the telephone lines or cable TV wires.
❒ Service provider	Also know as ISP (Internet Service Provider) and indicates a company that provides access to the Internet, usually for a monthly fee.
❒ Flame	The equivalent of yelling online in which the sender communicates disapproval or disagreement in very harsh language, often indicated by typing the message IN CAPS, LIKE THIS, for added emphasis
❒ Emoticons	An acronym for emotion icons; a small icon composed of punctuation characters that indicate the writer's mood. Emoticons need to be read sideways, as in this example for happy :-) or this one for yelling or shocked :-0; also called "smileys." For some great fun, go online to The Official Smiley Dictionary (*smileydictionary.com*) and try not to laugh as the yellow smiley-face chases your cursor around its homepage! Then have more fun learning much more than you ever wanted to know about this rather endearing Internet character!

In an undergraduate nursing course at Webster University (St. Louis, Missouri) called "Nursing and the Internet," Margo Thompson, Ed.D., R.N., provides the course objectives in the following list, which you could use as a guide to your own leaning about the Internet. You can access this syllabus at *webster.edu/~thompsma/internet/* and get a sense of what an online nursing course might look like, since online learning is quite likely to be in your future as the 21st century continues to unfold. Place a check mark next to the objectives that you believe you have already met, and then add a few more of your own:

❏ Describe Internet services

❏ Describe components of Web addresses

❏ Use search engines to find information on specific health and nursing topics

❏ Find and demonstrate ability to list and read messages in newsgroups and listservs related to health

❏ Send, read, forward, reply, save, and print email messages

❏ Connect to a medical library on the Internet and use publicly accessible resources

❏ Discuss issues related to evaluation of websites and the information they contain

❏ _____

❏ _____

❏ _____

For more information about distance learning, including a sampling of the University of Colorado nursing course, see Chapter 3, "The State of Nursing Education."

Learning More about the Internet

The following Internet sites are excellent resources for learning the basics, or to use when you are stumped. The process in which these sites were obtained provides a good example of how the Internet works. The steps are as follows:

Step 1: Using the AOL (America Online™) search engine, "define Internet terms" was typed in.

Step 2: A list of 36 Internet sites was returned. The site that was investigated had the Web address indicated below and was described as follows:

> *Internet terms:* Someone is always a mouse click away from helping you! The following is a short list of links that will help you define Internet terms: *coe.west.asu.edu/students/hcarter/internet_terms.htm*

Step 3: When this site was accessed, it not only provided the definitions of Internet terms but links to seven additional websites whose goal was to demystify the Internet. Two of these sites are:

- Webopedia   *webopedia.com*
- Learn the Net   *learnthenet.com*

Step 4: Additional Internet resource sites that were discovered included:

- NetLingua   *fun-with-words.com/net_lingua.html*

Internet Resources for 21st-Century Nurses

The Internet has become as important a tool to your nursing practice and in the management of your career as any of the traditional ones with which you might be more familiar. In the 20th century you could get by without it, relying on familiar printed books and resources. Not so in the 21st century. While books will never be replaced, nothing beats the speed at which you can access information from a kind of cyberspace library. You could never have this many print resources in your home, office, or any healthcare organization in which you work. Almost everything you were able to do before the availability of the Internet, you can do online.

In order to discuss the vast Internet resources that you need to be able to access, some categories of interest to nurses has been developed and appear in the section below, along with examples and some descriptions of what you might find in each category. This is not meant to be an all-inclusive list, but rather a sampling of what is available. The categories are:

- Professional practice
- Nursing research
- Nursing education
- Employment and career management
- Nursing community

There are two other important categories: For clinical practice refer to the beginning of this chapter, especially the resources used in the scenario about Ida and Sam. For self-care, refer to Chapter 16, "The Resilient Nurse: Self-Care Strategies" Further resources appear in the back of this book.

Professional Practice

There is a vast representation of national and international nursing organizations, associations and institutions to which you can connect and with whom you can interact to enhance your professional growth and track important professional practice issues.

One of the many ways to find voluminous lists of nursing and healthcare sites that match your professional needs and interests is to access the site of The American Nurses Association (ANA) (*nursingworld.org*). The ANA reports on national nursing issues, issues related to nursing practice, actions of government agencies, and so on. A recent issue of interest about which you could learn on the this site is the signing of the Nurse Reinvestment Act by President Bush on August 1, 2002, that authorizes federal funds to ease the nursing shortage. You can track the latest legislation passed or pending in different states by going to: *nursingworld.org*.

The ANA provides links to nursing, medical, health, and governmental sites of interest to nurses and others. There you will find lists of the websites listed below and be provided with direct links to each of these sites, which will link you to even more sites, forever onward into cyberspace:

- Academic organizations
- General nursing practice forums and institutes
- International nursing organizations
- Listservs and newsgroups
- Publications and references
- Specialty practice associations
- State boards of nursing index
- Tutorial and online continuing education

Other sites that will provide you with similar information are:

- Pennsylvania Nurses Association   *psna.org*
- New York State Nurses Association   *nysna.org/links.htm*
- *Nursing Spectrum*   *nursingspectrum.com*
- *Advance for Nurses*   *nursing.advanceweb.com/main.aspx*

Additional sites of interest to professional practice include:

- The National Institute of Health (NIH) *www.nih.gov,* which offers information about healthcare, research, grants available, data on diseases, clinical trials, and so on. Examples of what you might find on the NIH homepage include information about the West Nile Virus and hormone replacement therapy.

- The Centers for Disease Control (CDC) *www.cdc.gov* is the federal agency that protects the health and safety of people in the United States by monitoring health in the nation and in the world. Examples of what you would find on the CDC homepage includes the use of the smallpox vaccine and information about anthrax.

- The Food and Drug Administration (FDA) *www.fda.gov* is the federal agency that provides health and safety through the regulation of food, cosmetics, medical devices, and so on. An example of what you might find at this site includes information about buying medications online.

- The International Council of Nurses (ICN) *icn.ch/abouticn.htm* represents nurses from 120 countries. Its mission is to provide quality nursing practice and influence health policy. Issues of interest you will find at this site include AIDS and primary healthcare.

- The mission of the World Health Organization (WHO) *who.int/en* is to monitor the health needs of people worldwide. Health issues you will find on this site include communicable diseases, traveler health needs, and so on.

- The site of the American Medical Association (AMA) is *ama-assn.org.* Issues of relevance to nursing practice can often be found in JAMA, the *Journal of the American Medical Association*, including an important study about the nursing shortage conducted by Peter Buerhaus, Ph.D., R.N., of Vanderbilt University and his colleagues from Dartmouth that has been available to read online as of June 2002.

- To track licensure issues online, access the website of the National Council for State Boards of Nursing at *ncsbn.org.* Because each state has different nurse practice and regulation acts, this site will guide you through the use of its search engine to the state in which you require information.

- Nursing publications and references and journals of interest to nurses can be accessed at: *NursingNet.org.* Here you will find links to national and international journals, publications and reference tools, including the National Library of Medicine, *Medscape, Medline, The Merck Manual*, and many, many more.

Nursing Research

For news on research, abstracts, poster sessions, and other research-oriented information, access *nysna.org* and find the link to "nursing research." Other nursing associations will provide similar links. Also access Sigma Theta Tau, International Honor Society of Nursing (*nursingsociety.org*), and find the link to the Florence Henderson International Library. Dissertation abstracts are available online from many schools, including Barry University at *barry.edu/nursing/PHD/disertationAbstracts.htm*.

Nursing Education

Many colleges and universities are offering entire degrees online. Examples of these distance learning options are:

- The University of Phoenix offers the B.S.N. and M.S.N./M.B.A.: *uopxonline. com*.
- Jacksonville University School of Nursing offers an R.N. to B.S.N. program: *jacksonvilleu.com*.
- The State University of New York at Stony Brook offers an R.N. to B.S.N. program, M.S.N. programs and postmasters' certificate programs: *sonce1. nursing.sunysb.edu/nursingweb.nsf/aboutdistancelearning?openform*.
- The American Psychological Association (APA) format used almost universally for the writing and publication of papers can be accessed online at *apastyle.org*.
- For undergraduate nursing students preparing for the state board licensing exams, there are several test prep sites including *kaptest.com*. This site will also lead you to information about other tests, including the GRE, for those interested in applying to graduate schools.

For continuing education, often a requirement for relicensure and certification (differs from state to state), try these sites:

- The New York State Nurses Association   *nysna.org*
- Nursing Spectrum   *nursingspectrum.com*

Online in-service education, including "just in time" programs, are coordinated by an educational consortium and may be available in your place of employment. During the anthrax scare of 2001, nurses utilized "just in time" education provided by the CDC to learn the necessary protocols.

For additional information on nursing education, especially about distance learning, see Chapter 3, "The State of Nursing Education."

Employment and Career Management

Many local and national sites can be accessed to explore employment possibilities. Among them are:

- Monster.com   *monster.com*
- Nursing Spectrum   *nursingspectrum.com*
- The *New York Times*   *jobmarket.nytimes.com/pages/jobs*

Also try the home page/website of any healthcare organization in which you are interested in employment. Use search engines to locate the organizations of interest to you and then find their links to the Human Resources Department.

For assistance writing your resumes and cover letters:

- Career Journal   *jobstar.org*
- Monster.com   *resume.monster.com/writingservices/index.asp?msource=HP_V1*
- Kaplan Career Center   *kaptest.com*

For interview practice using virtual interview questions:

- Monster.com   *interview.monster.com/virtualinterview*
- For tips on how to prepare for job fairs   *jobsearch.about.com/library/blfairtip.htm*

Nursing Community

Three ways in which you can stay connected to colleagues in the local, national, and international nursing community are by utilizing listservs, usenet newsgroups, and chat rooms:

Listservs, also called email lists:

- *nurseweek.com*
- *nursingspectrum.com/nursecommunity/index.htm*

Specialized listservs include:

- *rnpalm.com/listserv.htm* for nursing information related to the personal digital assistant (PDA)
- *nursingworld.org* for lists of listservs maintained by the ANA

Usenet Newsgroups

These are available on Internet Service Providers such as America Online (AOL) and through any search engine by requesting a particular interest. For example, if you are a nursing student and want news related to the NCLEX-RN® exam, from any search engine, type in "NCLEX test prep" and among the many you will find listed there is the Kaplan Test Prep Center. Following the links, you will eventually be led to a site for *The Nursing Edge*, an email newsletter about the NCLEX-RN® exam and other information to plan and advance your nursing career.

Chat Rooms

Comprised of groups of people with common interests, chat rooms are ideal for talking in "real-time" with colleagues, when working on projects, and so on. Internet service providers that have active nursing chat rooms include America Online (AOL) and Microsoft Network (MSN). To find additional chat rooms, search for them by typing in "chat rooms" at any search engine.

THE INFORMATICS NURSE

A nursing role that has emerged in the last decade as the computer and Internet become omnipresent in healthcare is the informatics nurse. In 1994, the ANA defined the scope of practice for nursing informatics as a:

> ". . . combination of nursing science, computer science, and information science used in identifying, collecting, processing and managing data and information to support nursing practice, administration, education, research and the expansion of nursing knowledge."

The American Nurses Credentialing Center, the arm of the ANA that offers certification in many nursing specialties, offers certification for the informatics nurse who meets the following qualifications:

- Possess a bachelor's degree or higher
- Has at least two years of nursing practice experience as an R.N., with 2,000 hours of practice in nursing informatics
- Has attended at least 20 contact hours of continuing education in informatics nursing

Roles and responsibilities of the informatics nurse might include:

- Teach nurses how to research information on disease management
- Evaluate online patient education materials
- Evaluate and recommend software and hardware for providers and agencies
- Coordinate data from multiple sources
- Participate in research relevant to current trends in clinical information systems
- Participate on committees making decisions about new information technologies
- Participate in computer education for staff

The profile of Lt. Col. Florence Valley, R.N., an informatics nurse in the U.S. Air Force can be read online at *HospitalSoup.com/Day/nurse/ltcolvalley.asp*. There, you will be able to read what a typical day is like for this nurse, how her role differs from that of other nurses, what her educational preparation is, what she finds most enjoyable and most challenging, salaries for informatics nurses, and additional information as well.

Happy surfing!

CHAPTER 5

The Newly Graduated Nurse

WELCOME TO NURSING!

You are embarking on a career in which you will be offered a diversity of experiences and challenges that are among the finest opportunities for professional achievement and personal growth to be found anywhere.

You are entering the profession at a time of expanded opportunity as well as unprecedented challenges. While this is certainly a confusing time, it is also an exciting time, a time of turning points and crossroads, a time when some of the old ways restricting and inhibiting the image and value of nursing are beginning to fade away. This positive perception of the changes in nursing and healthcare can shape your purpose, your mission, your vision for yourself as a nurse, and sustain you through the challenges inherent in all worthwhile endeavors, and ultimately provide you with the professional satisfaction you are seeking.

Think back to the image you had of yourself as a nurse before entering nursing school, what you imagined you would be doing, how, where, and with whom. Now, fast-forward to the image you currently have of yourself. Is it the same? Different?

Most likely, the experiences you had and the people you met as you moved through your years of school have modified (without entirely changing) the ideal image you might have had, and replaced it with an image much closer to reality. This same process of moving from ideal to real is about to happen all over again as you leave the familiar nursing school community and enter the nursing practice arena. Your challenge will be to adapt to the reality of the work world without leaving all of your ideals and values behind.

You'll leave nursing school with a certain sense of mastery and proficiency about how to be a nursing student, along with an accumulation of knowledge that is in need of application in order to develop into the skills and competencies that will eventually define you as a nurse. In your first job, you will experience the emergence of your nursing identity, fragile at first, and hopefully protected and nurtured by the guidance and mentoring of those that came before you, while leaving enough space for your unique nursing personality to blossom.

THE JOURNEY FROM NOVICE TO EXPERT

To be a new graduate is to straddle two worlds, the recent past and the hopeful future, while maneuvering through what might feel like an obstacle course of learning challenges. You will be considered a novice, moving through five progressive stages that over many years, will eventually qualify you as an expert nurse. You might already be familiar with this learning model that was developed by Patricia Benner, R.N., Ph.D, F.A.A.N., and described in her book, *From Novice to Expert*.[1] Refreshing your memory about these important stages can reassure you about what to expect and provide you with guideposts that will help you chart your course and measure your progress. J. Mae Pepper, Ph.D., R.N. in her book, *Conceptual Bases of Professional Nursing* adapted Benner's five stages as follows on the next page.

BENNER'S STAGES FROM NOVICE TO EXPERT

	Stage I	Stage II	Stage III	Stage IV	Stage V
Title	Novice*	Advanced Beginner	Competent	Proficient	Expert
Experience level	Graduate*	New Graduate	2–3 years in the same setting	3–5 years	Extensive
Characteristics of performance	Is flexible	Formulates principles	Plans	Perceives "wholes"	Has an intuitive grasp
	Exhibits rule-governed behaviors	Needs help with priority-setting	Feelings of mastery	Interprets nuances	

* Stage I (the novice stage) occurs in nursing school. The newly graduated nurse begins nursing practice at Stage II, the advanced beginner.

Crucial to your ability to cope with the transition from student to nurse is an understanding of the timelines between Stage II, advanced beginner (the stage after nursing school when you enter nursing practice), and Stage V, (expert). While there are exceptions, the average time between stages is highlighted below:

- It takes 2–3 years in the same setting in order to achieve the competence of Stage III.
- It takes an additional year or so to achieve the proficiency of Stage IV.
- It takes an extensive and undetermined number of years to achieve the expert status of Stage V.[2]

Develop Realistic Expectations

Why is this important to understand and remember? I'll bet you're a good enough critical thinker to figure it out! Because every time you become impatient with yourself for not getting something right, every time you think you are taking too long to learn a complicated skill or procedure, or whenever you're convinced that you'll never be able to interpret cardiac arrhythmias fast enough, think back to this timeline, place yourself in it according to the years (not months!) you've been a nurse, and assess yourself accordingly.

The expectations you have of yourself as a new graduate and the kind of inner dialogue/self-talk (positive or negative) that accompanies them, will surely influence how you feel about yourself, as well as how effectively you will be able to master nursing skills and competencies. If your expectations are unrealistic—and holding yourself to a level of proficiency outside these timelines certainly qualifies as unrealistic—then, an obstacle of your own making has been created. Since plenty of obstacles already exist, it is unnecessary to create more of them, and cruel to yourself as well. Your emerging and vulnerable nursing identity requires better protection than that from you. Allowing yourself to be where you are, not where you wish you could be, combines self-care practice with professional nursing practice—one without the other neutralizes the effectiveness of both. Read more about this in Chapter 16, "The Resilient Nurse: Self-Care Strategies."

Dealing with the Expectations of Others

You might find that while your expectations are relatively realistic (or at least you are working in this direction), the expectations of some others around you are not. There might be impatience or criticism, or unhelpful comments or behaviors from established nurses or other healthcare personnel. New graduates (as well as novices everywhere) are very vulnerable to the opinions of others in their quest to belong and be accepted by their new peers and colleagues. This normal socialization process is part of your transition to practice and in many cases is quite enjoyable and invigorating.

While it is important to build this new professional community and keep it intact, this cannot be done at the expense of your emerging nursing identity. This presents you with a dilemma, one of many that you will likely come across, best solved with the assistance of someone, often a mentor, who can help you evaluate the veracity of the criticism. Every new graduate benefits from a relationship with someone who can provide this kind of essential reality check to ensure that the potentially inaccurate beliefs of others do not negatively influence the formation of your nursing identity. At the very minimum, a new graduate needs a preceptor, someone who acts as a clinical resource while you learn and practice basic nursing skills. Optimally, look for a way to have both a mentor *and* a preceptor. The preceptor will often be assigned to you as part of your orientation program. You may need to find the mentor on your own.

Seek Out a Mentor

A mentor is a guide, teacher, coach, counselor, advocate, role model, and nurturer; a person with whom you establish a personal, one-on-one relationship with the purpose of helping you to grow professionally and work toward your potential by means of:

- Obtaining feedback about your performance
- Setting and attaining goals, including identifying barriers to achieving them
- Developing plans for solving problems

The word *mentor* comes from the Greek legend of Odysseus who had a loyal friend and wise adviser whose name was Mentor. One of the best ways you can ensure that your transition from graduate to nurse has the support and nurturing it deserves is to find a mentor. It may take some self-directive, proactive, assertive activity on your part but it is worth your time and energy. There may be a faculty person who would be willing to mentor you or someone you met at a conference or CE seminar, or someone you have known through a listserv and have since met and with whom you have deepened your relationship. Or, it might be someone who taught in your orientation program. One consideration is to select someone who does not work on your unit so that you can speak more openly, with less fear of possible repercussions.

Nurses Nurturing Nurses (N3)

An additional way in which medical-surgical nurses may be able to find a mentor is through a new program in the process of being created by the Academy of Medical-Surgical Nurses called "Nurses Nurturing Nurses" (N3 for short). Since some organizations are acting as pilot sites for this new program, you might find yourself able to take advantage of it. Or, suggest that your organization contact the Academy to express their interest in participating. You can find out more as this exciting program evolves by logging on to their website: *medsurgnurse.org/cgi-bin/WebObjects/AMSNMain.woa*.

STRADDLING TWO WORLDS

New graduates straddle two worlds, the familiar world of nursing school and the exciting but rather intimidating world of nursing practice. Since they can inhabit only one of them, they must find a way to understand what is necessary to successfully move from one to the other.

Even though written in the last quarter of the 20th century, Marlene Kramer's seminal 1977 work, *Reality Shock* continues to have relevance to the 21st-century nurse in his or her struggle to leave the values of the school-world behind and adopt the values of the work-world, the nursing practice world. Reality shock happens when:

> " . . . newcomers in an occupational field find themselves in a work situation for which they have spent several years preparing and for which they thought they were going to be prepared, and then suddenly find that they are not."[3]

It soon becomes evident to this newcomer that the professional ideals and values he or she learned in school are not operational nor are they embraced or accepted by those in the workplace. It is this disparity in values that becomes a conflict requiring effective resolution if the newcomer is to transition successfully.

Kramer identifies four stages that new graduates will move through on their way to resolving the conflicts that are certain to emerge between the two worlds. The capacity for conflict management and resolution are essential to a successful transition. These stages are summarized below and like the Benner model, can provide you with another way to know what to expect, so that you can chart your course and measure your progress. The stages described below are adapted from Kramer's original work, and include the conflict likely to arise that will require successful resolution.

Stage I: **The Mastery of Skills and Routines**

Characteristics: There is a preoccupation with the development of technical expertise.

Potential conflict: Fixating on technical skills prevents sufficient focus on learning other aspects of nursing care such as teaching, emotional support, etc.

Stage II: **Social Integration**

Characteristics: Getting along with coworkers and being accepted by them is a major concern.

Potential conflict: Fear of retaliation and alienation may prevent the new graduate from applying knowledge learned in school.

Stage III:	Moral Outrage
Characteristics:	The new graduate feels frustrated and inadequately prepared.
Potential conflict:	The new graduate is confused about his or her role, and to what group or individual his/her loyalty belongs: the healthcare organization, the profession of nursing, or the patient.

Stage IV	Conflict Resolution
Characteristics:	Three possible outcomes:

1. Wholesale rejection of school culture and values leading to a kind of robotic adaptation to work values and behaviors accompanied by helpless resignation and the potential for burnout

2. Wholesale rejection of work culture and values leading to job-hopping in the hopes of finding a better match for the school values the new graduate is unwilling to give up; When job-hopping fails, these nurses typically leave the profession altogether

3. A joining of the school culture and the work culture in which the values from both represent a bicultural compromise solution that allows the new graduate to use the "best of both worlds" on behalf of the healthcare organization, the patient, and him/herself

STRATEGIES FOR SUCCEEDING

Now that you have a context in which to understand and track your experience, the following tips and strategies will assist you in transitioning successfully into nursing practice:

Celebrate Your Achievement

Begin your journey into nursing practice on a celebratory note. Sure, it's going to be a challenge, but nursing school was certainly a challenge to which you rose well enough to make nursing practice the next step in your career. Hooray for you! Do not forget this achievement; it will sustain you during your next challenges.

Select Your First Job Carefully

Choices abound; determine what the expectations will be of you, especially if, because of the nursing shortage, there is an unrealistic expectation for you to function as a nurse faster than you are able or is possible. Get the longest and best orientation possible. Be sure you will have a preceptor, perhaps even a mentor. Ask about the nurse-patient ratio and about overtime policies. Seek out healthcare organizations that have Magnet status certification for the best nursing practice environments. Refer to Chapters 1 and 2 for more information about this.

Extend Your Orientation

On your own, that is, after your formal orientation is over, keep it going in any self-directed way you can. Explore the continuing education programs in your organization, register for online CEs, and so on. Your graduation from nursing school signaled the continuation of your education, not the end of it.

Be the Best You Can Be

Be kind to yourself as a learner, allowing yourself the time it takes to gain proficiency. Recognize that learning occurs as a process that requires repetition. Forget perfect performance: it doesn't exist. Stay clear of a failing performance for obvious reasons. Aim for the middle ground. Perfect is too stressful and does not exist anywhere in the universe, including within you. Much of what you are learning requires practice, practice, practice, with a measured dose of patience, patience, patience.

Find a Mentor, Be a Mentor

Do you remember, "see one, do one"? Meaning, first you watch a task being done, then you do it as you've seen it. Think of mentoring in the same way. Find one, then be one. This is a time in nursing that the nurturing inherent in mentoring is needed by everyone. You don't have to wait to reach the expert level of proficiency to mentor others in something you are great at and they are not. Read the story of Ida and Sam in Chapter 4, "The Nurse and Technology," to see how they were mentors for one another. You might also want to mentor someone from high school who wants to be a nurse. What an important contribution to the nursing shortage you can make by doing this! Investigate the National Student Nurses' Association program called "Breakthrough to Nursing" to learn how to do this.

Seek Out Older Nurses

An experienced nurse can have a tremendous impact on your professional life and role development. Older nurses, nurses practicing at the expert level of proficiency have valuable wisdom and insights to impart. They are important clinical and professional resources. This person can often provide you with many decades of nursing history, the spoken, interactive kind you won't find in textbooks in quite the same way.

Be cautious about judgments or opinions you may have about their input or influence on such persistent nursing issues as relationships with physicians or the current nursing shortage. Recognize that the strength of the nursing profession is in its diversity, meaning the four generations of nurses currently practicing.

Believe in Yourself

Just because you're new, doesn't mean you can't make some amazing things happen. Become politically astute and develop the relationships required so that your ideas can have the influence and impact you desire.

Affirmations Really Do Work!

Ban negative thoughts or neutralize them with something positive. As soon as you hear yourself say something like, "I'll never learn this," be ready to banish it with some version of, "Every day, I am improving in my ability to _____" (fill in the blank for yourself).

Join a Support Group

Look for a new graduate support group in your organization and join it. Or, suggest that one gets formed. Seek out older nurses who are interested in providing this kind of experience and ask them to lead it. At the very minimum, go online to your favorite nursing listserv, newsgroup, or chat room and talk up a storm about what you are experiencing and hear what other nurses think about it, what they are doing. Remember that the stress of many experiences is relieved by the support of others with whom you can talk. You teach this to your patients, now use it for yourself.

CHAPTER **6**

The Second-Career Nurse

Enthusiastic. Focused. Mature. Motivated. Committed. Eager. Possessing a wealth of work and life experience.

These characteristics frequently describe the people that decide to make nursing a second career and who for a variety of reasons found themselves on a different life path when they were younger, perhaps keeping the flame of desire for nursing lit until a later time. When younger, someone might have dissuaded them from selecting nursing as a career, but as they matured they took another look for themselves. Or, they might have begun nursing studies and had to leave when something in their life required more of their attention. Since nursing is one of the professions in which it is possible to start a career in midlife, those who have had to wait often find that it is not too late.

Whatever the reason for the delay, what matters most is the fulfillment of these individuals' career goals as well as the idealism and contagious enthusiasm they can bring to the ranks of working nurses. It's invigorating to be in the presence of a nursing student who is finally achieving what he or she might have long planned and hoped for, or to be working alongside a second-career nurse who can provide a different and often refreshing perspective. During this time of difficulty resulting from the effects of the nursing shortage, this fresh spirit is welcome, indeed!

TWO GREAT REASONS FOR BECOMING A NURSE

If you are a second-career nurse reading this chapter, congratulations for making this important life decision! (Have you considered recruiting friends?) If you are someone considering nursing as a second career, read on! The nursing profession needs you. While you are certainly entering nursing at a challenging time for the profession, there are two reasons not to let this stop you. The first is that all challenges are opportunities in disguise, crucibles for growth, and pathways to immense personal and professional satisfaction.

The second reason to say yes to nursing as your second career is that you just may be in the right place at the right time! Financial assistance is about to become a plentiful enticement that could easily make this decision easier than you thought. At the time this book was being published, Congress had just passed a funding bill called the Nurse Reinvestment Act in order to ease the nursing shortage. Among the ways in which you can track the progress and availability of this funding online is at the website of your state nurses association—listed at the back of this book—as well as at the website of the American Association of Colleges of Nursing *www.aacn.nche.edu.*

For those of you who are already nurses, second career or otherwise, don't think you've missed the financial boat! Consider using the financial assistance that is about to be more available than ever to advance your education. For a more complete discussion of the multitude of options available for you to begin or advance your nursing education, either in the many traditional or the newly emerging virtual classrooms of online distance learning, consult Chapter 3, "The State of Nursing Education." You will also find print and online resources in the Resources to guide you in your decision.

NURSING IS MUCH MORE THAN A JOB

For many nurses, whether this is their first or second career, nursing represents more than just a job, even more than a career—it is a calling. It taps a deep inner well of desire to contribute something meaningful, to make a difference. Many nurses describe being recommitted to the spirit of caring that is the essence of nursing following the devastating events of September 11ᵗʰ.

A typical response of many people to that momentous day was a reevaluation of their goals and priorities, including the desire to be engaged in something meaningful.

This is what nurses have the opportunity to do everyday. Listen to the words of Melissa Velazquez, a staff nurse on the burn intensive care unit at Washington Hospital Center in Washington, DC, as described by Susan Trossman, R.N. in "Nurses Share Accounts of 9-11 Aftermath" (*The American Nurse*, November/December 2001):

> "Nurses will drop everything they are doing to go where they are needed. Altruism is at the core of nursing. It's who we are."[1]

You can read the full account of Melissa Velazquez's experience and the inspiring accounts of other nurses as well by accessing the article online at *nursingworld.org/tan/ 01novdec/aftermat.htm*. The article ends with suggestions of how nurses can help, along with a link (*geocities.com/Heartland/Woods/6780*) to the stories of the nine nurses who lost their lives as a result of the attacks on September 11th.

To read the outstanding contribution made by the nursing faculty and their students at several New York schools of nursing on September 11th, as well as additional stories of how nurses participated on that day or in the aftermath, access "Stories from the Field" at *nysna.org/*.

WHO CHOOSES NURSING AS A SECOND CAREER?

In "Finding Their Way" by Mary Ann Hellinghausen (*Nurse Week*, December 6, 1999, *nurseweek.com*), Edwards Russell, Ph.D., R.N., head of th nursing department and an associate professor at Angelo State University, says the following about the second-career nurse: "They often are strongly driven. They understand client needs—the need to take care of their patients. They know nursing is a very client-focused profession."[2]

Nursing is an attractive option to many people seeking meaningful work. Those who choose nursing as a second career often have the characteristics or experiences described below and on the next page. Check the ones that most closely describe you or what you are seeking in a career.

❑ People who are transferring or retiring from other service industries such as fire fighters and police officers, or healthcare workers such as emergency medical technicians; Typically these people still desire the stimulation of a fast-paced environment linked with the satisfaction of helping others but want to experience it in a new venue

❏ People, often other healthcare workers, who have worked alongside registered nurses as nursing assistants, unit secretaries, or social workers

❏ People who are feeling unfulfilled and disillusioned by their work in the business world or in other industries, and who are seeking more meaning in their lives

❏ People whose family or financial responsibilities no longer preclude their ability to focus on their career goals

❏ People who are seeking the relative job security that nursing represents, even in this age of managed care and economic restraint; As long as a nurse remains flexible in skills, competencies, and most important, attitude, he or she will always find work

❏ People who want the stimulating combination of high tech and high touch; While some nurses prefer low tech rather than high tech practice settings, "no tech" is not an option for any nurse

❏ People who are seeking comparatively good salaries, at least at the entry level, although whether salaries are high enough is debatable among practicing nurses

❏ People who enjoy the challenge and stimulation of healthcare's constant learning environment, of incorporating what's new and what's next into their work, as science and technology continue to wage war against disease and injury

❏ People seeking to utilize a broad skill base; The Bureau of Labor Statistics identifies eight universal skills in its 2002–3 *Occupational Outlook Handbook (www.bls.gov);* Nursing uses all of them (See chart on following page.) These are:
   ❏ Leadership/persuasiveness
   ❏ Helping/instructing others
   ❏ Problem solving/creativity
   ❏ Initiative
   ❏ Work as part of a team
   ❏ Frequent public contact
   ❏ Manual dexterity
   ❏ Physical stamina

❏ Smart people who recognize the vast career options and flexibility of nursing careers

Skills for Success

The U.S. Bureau of Labor Statistics lists eight "universal" job skills in its *Occupational Outlook Handbook*. Nursing requires all eight skills.

Selected list of professions	Leadership/ persuasiveness	Helping/ instructing others	Problem solving/ creativity	Initiative	Work as part of a team	Frequent public contact	Manual dexterity	Physical stamina
Registered nurses	●	●	●	●	●	●	●	●
LPNs/LVNs		●			●	●	●	●
Physicians		●	●	●	●	●	●	
Pharmacists	●	●	●	●	●	●	●	
Lab techs		●			●		●	
Social workers	●	●		●	●	●		
Psychologists		●	●	●		●		
Sociologists			●	●		●		
Air traffic controllers		●	●	●	●		●	
Pilots			●	●	●		●	
Architects			●	●	●	●	●	
Biological scientists			●	●				
Priests/rabbis/ ministers	●	●	●	●	●	●		
Correction officers	●	●			●			●
Construction workers			●		●		●	●
Accountants and auditors		●	●		●	●		
Actors, directors, and producers			●	●	●	●	●	●

Healthcare is a growth industry; nursing is the largest profession in healthcare and offers a wide choice of employment settings, along with a continuum of care that includes health maintenance as well the care of those ill or injured, of all ages, and in a multitude of medical specialties. Only burnout can prevent a nurse from having a long, satisfying, and stimulating career considering the professional diversity that is available. See Chapter 11, "The Market Research Department of *You, Inc.*" for a more complete description of the vast career options from which nurses can choose.

PROFILES OF TWO SECOND-CAREER NURSES

Tim Hein, a 45-year-old nursing student

In "One Solution to Nursing Shortage: Second-Career Trainees" by Nicholas Engels (*The Business Journal of Milwaukee, milwaukee.bizjournals.com*), Tim Hein, a 45-year-old registered nursing student talks about his experiences, saying, "People in nursing are by nature helpful; some students don't stick around long enough to realize that." Last year Tim felt he needed to enter an industry with the opportunity to pursue a hands-on leadership role.

Tim wanted a more versatile degree than the first one he got in healthcare management and so chose nursing. It was the influence of his girlfriend, a nurse, that convinced him it was a good avenue to pursue, even though he wouldn't have considered it 20 years ago.

Tim believes the merits of nursing as a second career far outweigh the adversities he faces each day. He says:

> "Like anything, nursing takes time. Going back to school is tough, but as a rule, both teachers and students are a helpful group of people. That makes the transition a lot smoother."[3]

Dwight Simmons, M.B.A., B.S.N., R.N., a medical-surgical nurse on a liver transplant unit

In "Second Sight," by Rose Quinn in *Advance for Nurses* (July 22, 2002, *nursing.advanceweb.com/main.aspx*), you will find the story of Dwight Simmons, who at age 50 has worked as a nurse for three years and embodies many of the characteristics of second-career nurses. Dwight was an optician for 22 years before he made the transition to nursing which began seven years ago after administering vocational tests to himself and discovering that nursing was one of four careers best suited to him. The others were physician, mortician, and optician. Becoming a nurse, he says, was not a matter of settling. His wife supported the decision and thought he would be great at it.

Dwight correctly assessed the field to be wide open even though he began nursing school, part-time at first, in 1995 at the height of the downsizing and restructuring era in healthcare. Since he already had a degree in biology, he needed only to take the nursing courses, receiving credit for about half of the requirements needed to complete his B.S.N. He also has an M.B.A. in marketing and one day hopes to follow his nurse manager's (and mentor's) footsteps into management. His vision of himself five years from now includes a master's degree in nursing administration and advanced learning in information systems.

For now, Dwight is quite content with his experience as a medical-surgical nurse on a liver transplant unit. While there has been some surprise and concern about his gender from a few of his patients, it is clear that Dwight's comfort with his identity as a nurse eventually puts the patients at ease, while he also models the kind of gender-neutral attitude that nursing needs to embrace among both women and men who are nurses. (For a discussion about the role of men in nursing, refer to Chapter 8, "Men: The Changing Face of Nursing.")

Dwight has the following to say about his experiences of being a nurse:

> "One of the greatest thrills is when someone comes back to the hospital months later. Sometimes you don't recognize them. You start to cry because they look so wonderful. It makes it all worthwhile . . . Being a nurse has given me a better appreciation of life."[4]

Dwight Simmons is certainly on his way to making important contributions to nursing and healthcare. It is clear that he is happy with the decision he made and is someone whom those seeking a second career in nursing could model themselves after.

TIPS FOR SECOND-CAREER NURSES

Getting Started

- Keep in mind that to ease the nursing shortage, schools and colleges of nursing are actively recruiting many underrepresented segments of the nursing profession, including men, minorities, and those seeking a second career as a nurse.

- Look for programs with flexible academic and clinical schedules so that you will be able to accommodate your current needs and responsibilities. Two colleges of nursing that have programs specifically designed for second career nurses are Marquette University in Wisconsin (*mu.edu*) and the University of Wisconsin at Milwaukee (*uwm.edu*). Many schools offer combined B.S.N./M.S. programs to applicants with a bachelor's degree in another field.

- See Chapter 3, "The State of Nursing Education," for additional information on how to select the program that is right for you.

In Nursing School

- Give yourself time to adapt to the rigorous academic and clinical learning environment in nursing school. While all students need to adjust to this, second-career students who may have prior college experience may not be prepared for the challenging intensity of nursing education. Nursing school is difficult and it should be. While communicating caring concern is a foundation of nursing practice, there's much more to being a nurse than this. Learning the science of nursing, how it differs from medicine, as well as mastering such courses as pathophysiology and pharmacology, and then applying what you are learning in clinical settings is challenging. Doable, but challenging, none the less.

- Handle the age gap that will most likely exist between you and other students who could be 10 to 20 or more years younger than you, depending on your own age.

- To access support and information while in nursing school, use the many wonderful student nurse communities you can find online. One of these is the National Student Nurse Association (*www.nsna.org*).

In Nursing Practice

- Practice balancing the priorities of your work life and your personal life. Refer to Chapter 16, "The Resilient Nurse: Self-Care Strategies" for information about why this kind of self-care is essential rather than incidental to your nursing practice.

- Temper your enthusiasm with respect and understanding for the first-career nurses with whom you will work side-by-side, since this is how you will want to be treated as well. Before judging what you may not understand, familiarize yourself with the historic and contemporary influences that impact and shape the variety of responses and behaviors of the profession as well as its individual members. A discussion of this can be found in Chapter 8, "Men: The Changing Face of Nursing."

Above all, dive in! Make a difference! And, *welcome*!

CHAPTER 7

The Older Nurse

What are we to call those legions of nurses edging near to retirement age, whose anticipated exodus is referred to again and again as contributing to the nursing shortage? What would be politically correct? Should they be called mature nurses? Or, do we call them elders? What about Boomers? Or, just older?

As the old (no pun intended!) saying goes, "call me anything, just don't call me late for the shortage"—the nursing shortage, that is. There could be a significant influence on the nursing shortage if these nurses were kept in the action or called back again as resources to support, educate, precept, and mentor those nurses entering the profession, as well as to provide direct patient care, as desired and feasible.

The following sobering statistics should sound alarm bells that result in immediate attention and swift action:

- The present average age of employed registered nurses is 43.3 years, with registered nurses who are under 30 years old representing only 10 percent of the total nursing workforce. (National League for Nursing, *www.nln.org*)

- In 2010, 40 percent of working R.N.s will be 50 years old or older; as those R.N.s retire, the supply of working R.N.s is projected to be 20 percent below requirements by the year 2020 (Peter Buerhaus, Ph.D, R.N., 6/14/00, *Journal of the American Medical Association*).

- Since 1995, nursing baccalaureate-level education rates have dropped 23 percent, and associate-level graduation rates have fallen 30 percent (National League for Nursing, *nln.org*). While a 3.7 increase in baccalaureate-level enrollment occurred in fall 2001, it is too soon to tell if this represents a significant upward trend.

- The average age of new R.N. graduates is 31. They are entering the profession at an older age and will have fewer years to work than nurses traditionally have had (Bureau of Labor Statistics, *www.bls.gov*).
- It is anticipated that the demand for nurses will outstrip the supply by 2010. (See chart in Chapter 2.)

Every statistic points not only to an aging workforce, but to one that will continue to be older than in previous generations, and at a time in history when the demands for healthcare will be greater than ever before.

RETAIN OLDER NURSES?

There are two populations of people at risk as a result of the nursing shortage: American citizens and nurses themselves. Both groups will suffer unless creative solutions to the nursing shortage are found. Americans will have substandard healthcare and a shrinking number of less experienced nurses will work under greater stress and enormous pressure in an attempt to care for them.

As in all crisis situations, of which the nursing shortage certainly qualifies, opportunities abound, waiting to be tapped in order to alter or improve the situation, in this case the stability of the profession as well as the nurses in it.

The retention of older nurses in the workforce is a strategy worth exploring since it is evident that the loss of their expertise through attrition and retirement will occur faster than replacements can be recruited and educated. Whether these nurses want to continue working and in what capacity are two of the many questions to be answered before retention can be addressed. Nursing associations, healthcare organizations as well as individual nurse-leaders are currently exploring this territory and making recommendations to accommodate the needs of older nurses. Some of their ideas and concerns appear in the next section, along with websites for you to track the progress of this important issue as it unfolds.

The American Nurses Association (ANA) at their 2002 convention passed a resolution (*nursingworld.org*) to address the "implications of the mature/experienced workforce." The ANA supports the following points of action:

- Heighten awareness of the critical need for the mature/experienced nurse to remain a core contributing professional
- Recommend mechanisms that would support the retention of mature/experienced nurses
- Advocate for the development of strategies that support the choice of the mature/experienced nurse to continue practicing and remain professionally active while recognizing the contribution of those who choose to retire
- Advocate that the institutional knowledge of the mature/experienced nurse be preserved and that the specialized nurse be retained
- Monitor the issues associated with the aging general workforce of Americans[1]

Peter Buerhaus, Ph.D, R.N., the Valere Potter Professor of Nursing at Vanderbilt University School of Nursing speaks about the needs of older nurses in "Wanted: A Few Good Nurses: Addressing the Nation's Nursing Shortage" by Barbara A. Gabriel in *AAMC Newsroom Reporter* (*www.aamc.org/newsroom/reporter/march01/nursing.htm*). Buerhaus says:

> ". . . a more mature workforce will have higher expectations of working conditions and demand greater autonomy in professional practice, issues that hospital administrators will need to be sensitive to in order to keep their more seasoned healthcare workers."[2]

The issue of ergonomics as well as other enticements and retention strategies for the older nurse was discussed by Pamela Thompson, executive director of the American Organization of Nurse Executives in "Experts Weigh-in on Issue of Retaining Older OR Nurses," (*Healthcare Purchasing News Online, hpnonline.com*) by Jane Martinsons. Thompson advocates for the following initiatives:

- Ask older nurses what they want.
- Offer flexible scheduling to allow more control over their lives.
- Balance the wishes of older nurses against those of their counterparts so that you don't create a retention strategy for one population in your workforce that then alienates another.
- Be aware of older nurses' physical limitations; focus on ergonomics: lessen the lifting strains that are likely to occur through technology or assistant personnel.

- Recognize older nurses' achievements through such incentives as clinical ladders and increased salaries.
- Offer in-site childcare and ill childcare programs for children or grandchildren.[3]

In "Staying Power" by Cathryn Domrose (*NurseWeek, nurseweek.com*), Leah Curtain, R.N., Sc.D., F.A.A.N., a Cincinnati, Ohio, researcher of nursing issues, discussed what she says older nurses want, according to her research. These include ergonomic improvements (better lighting, bigger print, etc.), flexible schedules, cross-training and continuing education, and a broader interpretation of family leave time that allows for the care of their ailing parents. In this same article, Jill Furillo, R.N., director of government relations for the California Nurses Association, spoke of her organization being successful in retaining older nurses by negotiating contracts that designated some as "resource nurses," working specifically as preceptors to younger nurses rather than squeezing in this responsibility among other duties related to providing direct care.[4]

In "Elder Nurses Tapped to Combat Shortage" by Ronni Sayewitz (*South Florida Business Journal, southflorida.bizjournals.com*) focus groups are among the strategies being used by Baptist Health South Florida to explore ways to meet the needs of mature nurses, which it defines as those over age 45. Eighty to 100 older nurses are expected to volunteer for these focus groups to express their opinions about the changes in job requirements that are being explored. These include shifts shorter than 12 hours, flexible schedules, and assigning patients within small areas to reduce the need for walking long distances. Additional initiatives at this organization include allocating budget funds for the purchase of new technology and resources that can ease the physical strain of nursing tasks. They are planning to replace their beds with ones that convert into chairs, store supplies and drugs closer to patients rooms to reduce the amount of walking, and hire more aides to perform strenuous duties like turning or lifting patients. Cathy Allman, the VP of nursing and healthcare professions, summarizes the ideas of this organization in a way that echoes the loud, insistent message being transmitted across the nation throughout the nursing and healthcare communities:

"Mature nurses bring experience and expertise you can't put a price on. If you can figure out a way to retain the good quality nurses in your organization, you won't have a shortage problem."[5]

MYTHS AND STEREOTYPES

One barrier to retaining the older nurse are the myths and stereotypes that inhibit older people from full participation in work in all industries. Aside from whether older nurses want to be retained in the workforce is the issue of American society's youth obsession with its accompanying attitude about older people/nurses. Reflect on the following statements and determine if you believe them to be true or false.

    ❐ True ❐ False   Older nurses are rigid and not open to change.

    ❐ True ❐ False   Older nurses are not good with technology and computers; they are not interested in them and don't like to learn about them.

    ❐ True ❐ False   Older nurses can't use critical thinking well and that makes them a hazard in today's fast-paced healthcare environments.

    ❐ True ❐ False   Older nurses are more prone to illness and call in sick more often.

    ❐ True ❐ False   Older nurses would not make good mentors, preceptors, or role models because they are too domineering and overbearing.

    ❐ True ❐ False   Older nurses have stopped caring; they're burned out and just cruising along, putting in their time.

Not only are all these statements false, they could just as easily be said about the younger generations of nurses. It is possible that these myths and stereotypes could lose some of their sting and negative influence by finding ways to keep older nurses in the workforce, utilizing the resources they have to offer. The nursing profession could lead the way and join other enlightened industries and workplaces in breaking down these 20th-century attitudes that no longer fit 21st-century lives.

The challenge in this nursing shortage is broader than the retention of the older nurse. The bigger challenge is not only to preserve the existing workforce, but also to improve the conditions in which *all* nurses work in order to prevent the problems associated with recruitment and retention from contributing to this kind of shortage in the future. This would benefit *all* nurses, young and old, alike.

FOUR GENERATIONS OF THE NURSING WORKFORCE

Rather than speaking of older and younger nurses, it seems more accurate to speak of four generations of nurses represented in the workforce. While authorities vary in what to call these generations and in what time span they were born, Carolyn Martin, a specialist in multigenerational issues affecting the workforce, discusses the following categories in her book, *Managing Generation Y*:

- *The Silent Generation*, born between 1925 and 1942
- *The Baby Boomers*, born between 1943 and 1962
- *Generation X*, born between 1963 and 1977
- *Generation Y*, born after 1978

The characteristics of these four generations are discussed by Cathryn Domrose in "Bridges Across Time" (*NurseWeek*, 5/14/01, *nurseweek.com*), and can be summarized as follows:

- *The Silent Generation* (also called the *GI Generation*)
   —Helped rebuild the American economy after World War II
   —Strong sense of commitment, loyalty, and hard work

- *The Baby Boomers*
   —Grew up pampered
   —Share workplace values of Silent Generation, including loyalty and commitment
   —Many went into nursing to "do good" in the world
   —Those who survived the downsizing of the '80s and '90s were forced to rely on each other to work overtime and cover shifts

- *Generation X* and *Generation Y*
   —Grew up as latchkey kids, in the era of downsizing and restructuring
   —Don't understand the fuss about overtime and overwork, pensions and retirement plans
   —Believe job security is a myth and that their best chance of survival in a changing workplace lies in building and marketing their skills
   —Work hard and are dedicated to their patients
   —Want to be paid adequately and are not afraid to tell employers when they think demands are unreasonable

These intergenerational characteristics of the nursing workforce create important issues to address, especially in the context of the reorganization of nursing roles and responsibilities being advocated by many nursing leaders as a strategy to utilize older nurses. The similarities between the generations are reassuring, while the differences highlight the areas of potential conflict that astute nurses and the organizations for which they work could identify to implement programs to increase awareness and manage conflicts. This could lessen the potential for interpersonal stress in a workforce already under significant pressure.

Each of these generations in nursing has much to teach the other, as did Sam and Ida in Chapter 4, "The Nurse and Technology," who mentored one another in their respective areas of expertise. Ida benefited from Sam's technology and computer abilities, while Sam, a new graduate, was able to learn nursing skills and competencies under Ida's expert tutelage and reassuring presence.

PROFILES OF OLDER NURSES

While Ida and Sam are fictional composites of real nurses, the following are profiles of actual nurses who remain active and contributing members of the nursing workforce:

Marie Cronk, age 61, and Rosalee Yeaworth, age 71, are two nurses profiled in "Gray Matters" by Ed Frauenheim in *NurseWeek* (*nurseweek.com/news/features/01-01/mature.asp*). Marie Cronk is a charge nurse and certified operating room nurse at Good Samaritan Hospital in Puyallup, WA, who told Freuenheim:

> "Experience is invaluable. I feel I have a lot of knowledge and I'm able to use it. And I try to pass it on to the younger people."

She speaks of maintaining her physical stamina through her commitment to exercising on her treadmill and a healthy diet.

Rosalee Yeaworth is a retired dean of the University of Nebraska Medical Center, College of Nursing and agreed to teach an Internet course in nursing theory when a faculty member at the college was unable to. She remarked:

> "I went back into teaching last fall not because I needed the money, but because the college needed help. It was stimulating to go back."[6]

Marilyn McMahon, age 55, is an emergency room nurse at Forest General Hospital in Hattiesburg, MS. What makes the profile of this nurse especially interesting is that she works at the same hospital as her three daughters, also nurses. Their profiles, which appear in "Bridges Across Time" by Cathryn Domrose (*NurseWeek*, 5/14/01, *nurseweek.com*), allow a peek into what nurses of different generations can offer one another as well as what an older nurse still at work might be doing.[7]

OLDER NURSES HAVE CHOICE

As the discussion about older nurses widens, as it surely will, you are likely to see additional profiles of what older nurses are doing, or choosing not to do, as the case may be. It is important to ensure that older nurses have a choice about their continued participation in the nursing workforce and that the strategies being developed recognize that choice in order to prevent the potential harassment and/or exploitation that might otherwise occur. One of the statements in the ANA resolution about the mature workforce discussed earlier in this chapter is worth repeating here:

> "Advocate for development of strategies that *support the choice* of the mature/experienced nurse to continue practicing and remain professionally active *while recognizing the contribution of those who choose to retire.*"

MAJOR MESSAGES FOR OLDER NURSES

Choose If and When You Want to Continue Working

Then, accurately assess your physical, mental, emotional, spiritual, and personal stamina. Be realistic about what you can and cannot do.

If You Choose Not to Continue Working

Celebrate your nursing achievements and accomplishments. Moving on to other experiences following a nursing career is just as important a decision as continuing to work, as long as it is a conscious choice made after deliberating and reflecting on your options.

Reassess Your Nursing Skills and Competencies

Determine how you want to continue using them. Watch for the options that healthcare organizations will be offering to older nurses and find a match between what they are offering and your reassessed skills and competencies. For example, if you are a critical care nurse who no longer desires to provide direct patient care, watch for mentoring, precepting, or teaching opportunities that do not require you to have your own patient care assignment.

Make Sure Your Voice Is Heard

Your opinions count heavily here. Healthcare organizations are gearing up to develop strategies to recruit and retain you in the workforce. Make sure they know what you need to make that happen, such as flexible hours, and so on. Be sure to maintain your professionalism by being realistic in your requests; look for win-win options that benefit you *and* the organization.

Be Part of the Dialogue

Track the discussion about this important issue any way you can. Go to conferences, read nursing journals and newsletters, and of course, get online and "hear" what others are saying and doing. Log on to the Academy of Medical-Surgical Nurses website (*medsurgnurse.org/cgi-bin/WebObjects/AMSNMain.woa*) to find out about their new mentoring program called "Nurses Nurturing Nurses," N3 for short.

Keep Current

Stay informed clinically and about current issues in the profession, and in healthcare. The best way to stay current is to use several websites and/or listservs, especially the American Nurses Association *(nursingworld.org)* or your state nurses' association. Refer to Chapter 4, "The Nurse and Technology" or the Resources for this information.

Provide Wisdom, Not Warnings

In your mentoring and preceptor relationships be sure you are sharing what's right and great about nursing, how far we've come, and where we still need to go. Share the lessons learned and the progress made. There is reason for optimism, even when the challenges are great. If you have trouble believing this, if you are of the opinion that "things never change," reconsider if mentoring is the right choice for you. This is not a time for doom and gloom thinking. If you must tell your war stories, tell them with a balanced perspective of then versus now, and consider including a healthy dose of humor.

Self-Care Really Counts Now!

This is especially true for physical self-care. Whatever you were able to get away with when you were younger is no longer possible. This is the truth! Believe it! If you want to stay a contributing member of the nursing community as well as the *human* community, take your self-care seriously. This means healthy eating, adequate exercise, and sufficient rest. Refer to Chapter 16, "The Resilient Nurse: Self-Care Strategies," for information on this, or to any resource that will motivate you to take charge of this essential part of your life.

Yours Is the Past, the Present, and the Future

Just as new graduates straddle the two worlds between school and work, so do older nurses straddle the worlds between two centuries, the 20th and the 21st, the time between old and new, between past and present. For those of you who choose to stay on in nursing, you have an opportunity to influence the world of nursing yet to be, the future. Yours is an opportunity to contribute in ways you might not have imagined five or ten years ago.

Your journey as a nurse may not be over yet. You may want to consider allowing it to continue longer for the benefit of other nurses who will follow in your footsteps and for those for whom they will care. After all, isn't the opportunity to make a difference to others why you became a nurse to begin with?

CHAPTER 8

Men: The Changing Face of Nursing

In this age of increasing tolerance for ethnic diversity and an ever-growing awareness of the damaging effect of gender barriers, that nursing is still a profession comprised 95 percent of women should raise a red flag of concern. This is especially true if the profession's current difficulty attracting people (women and men alike) is contributing to a risk in meeting the healthcare needs of American society. The National Advisory Council on Nursing Education and Practice warns that if nursing, which represents the largest healthcare profession, is to successfully address the unique needs of this country's growing minority populations, it is vital that they attract more men and minority groups.

> "Today men are resuming their historical role as caring, nurturing nurses, just as some women are resuming their roles as physicians. After a century as a predominantly female profession, nursing is changing again. It will be interesting to see what happens in the next century."
>
> —*Men in American Nursing History,* Bruce Wilson, R.N., Ph.D. *(b-wilson.net)*[1]

The shortage of nurses facing us today is a crisis and like all crises offers opportunities for something new and different to happen, including the possibility of something better. The presence of men in a profession long dominated by women may well represent something better, indeed.

Attracting more men into nursing is certainly not the only answer to the nursing shortage, or to ensuring America's healthcare needs. And, clearly, nursing's 95 percent female professionals are not waiting for, nor do they need to be "rescued" from their current difficulties by men. However, increasing the diversity, gender included, of any group of people has been shown to have positive effects on its culture, once barriers to diversity are identified and eliminated. There is every reason to believe this to be true for the culture of nursing as well. Interestingly, however, while nursing has made some inroads to increasing its cultural diversity, the same cannot be said of its gender mix.

THE GLASS GATE?

Some of what is experienced by men today seeking to become nurses or already working as nurses is reminiscent of what women experienced and are still experiencing as they enter male-dominated professions in healthcare, especially when they aim high and find themselves blocked by the so-called "glass ceiling." If women experience a "glass ceiling," do men entering nursing experience a "glass gate"? Why does the gate exist? What experiences do men have trying to get through it? What are some strategies for opening this gate that are successfully being used by individuals, institutions, and organizations? Who are the men that have succeeded in getting to the other side? How will the nursing profession and the healthcare industry benefit from the presence of more men?

The sections that follow begin to address these questions and ask others. You are invited to add your own answers to these questions, to think of additional questions, and to ask these questions among your professional and personal networks in order to increase awareness and generate solutions that can open wide the "glass gate."

WHY THE GLASS GATE EXISTS

In their *Issues Bulletin* (December 2001), the American Association of Colleges of Nursing (*www.aacn.nche.edu*) identified the following reasons men and minority group members do not pursue nursing:

- Role stereotypes
- Economic barriers
- Few mentors
- Gender biases
- Lack of direction from early authority figures

- Misunderstanding about the practice of nursing
- Increased opportunities in other fields[2]

Michael Williams, R.N., M.S.N., C.C.R.N., is the first male president of the American Association of Critical Care Nurses. In "President's Notes: A Journey of Rediscovery—So How Does it Feel to You?" (AACN News, August 2001, *aacn.org*), he identified the following "host of challenges" facing men who choose nursing:

- Invisibility
- Negative stereotypes
- Few male faculty members in nursing schools
- Male students socialized to downplay their gender
- Little opportunity to work and communicate with other men in nursing
- Misperceptions about our competence and qualifications for promotion
- Differences in how each gender communicates
- Perceptions that physicians automatically respect men in nursing more than women
- And, perhaps the most devaluing of all, the perception that a man cannot be caring and compassionate enough to be a nurse[3]

ROLE STEREOTYPES AND GENDER BIASES

The student leaders of the National Student Nurses Association (NSNA) recognize that interesting men in nursing requires male as well as female role models. In a question and answer column called "Breakthrough to Nursing" (*Imprint*, February/March 2002), Ashleigh Williams and Nikki Battle encourage "those participating in 'Breakthrough to Nursing' projects, particularly in elementary schools, to ensure that those representing nursing are a diverse group that include men."[4]

The idea that women become nurses and men become physicians is so deeply entrenched in the American psyche that as recently as July 2002, an article in a nursing publication which discussed nurse-physician relationships showed a drawing of a man in a white coat, pounding his fist in anger to make a point to a woman in casual professional dress with her arms folded across her chest. There was no caption under the picture, leaving it to the reader to decide who was the nurse and who was the physician. This was not difficult since the article used feminine pronoun "she" when referring to the nurse and the masculine pronoun "he" when referring to the physician. Would it have been illuminating or confusing if in the article "she" referred to the physician and "he" to the nurse? In what way might nursing, and the media be responsible for reinforcing the myth and stereotypes that become glass gates?

Among today's 5 percent, men who are currently nurses, there are some impressive role models. Michael Desjardins, R.N., the first male president of the National Student Nurses' Association, is one of them. He represents someone who succeeded in getting through the gate and is now in a position to influence how others might do so as well. In an article called "Looking for a Few Good Men" by Debra Williams (*Minority Nurse*, Spring 2002, *MinorityNurse.com*), Desjardins critiques a popular movie, a comedy called *Meet the Parents*, in which the actor Ben Stiller is seeking to marry a woman whose parents do not approve of him for many reasons, most particularly because he is a male nurse, the basis of many jokes throughout the movie. In this article Desjardins discusses how he knows too well that these fictional jokes are the reality for men who have chosen nursing as a career. He states, "After all of the chaos [Stiller's character causes], the one thing the father can't forgive is that he is a male nurse. I don't see that as funny." Williams states:

> "Desjardins confronts stereotypes about male nurses practically every day. People act surprised when they learn his occupation. Friends have told him to wear his wedding ring to work so people won't assume he's gay. Even though he's only been an R.N. for a year, Desjardins is already concerned about the effects his gender may have on his career path."[5]

This last statement should ring alarm bells for everyone in healthcare who is seeking to solve the nursing shortage, who cares about the future of nursing, and wants to ensure quality care for American people.

THE PUBLIC'S IMAGE OF NURSES

What the public thinks of the nurse in terms of appearance, perceived functions, prestige, and what they hear nurses say (or don't hear, as the case may be) ultimately determines the perceived value of nursing as a career choice. That nursing is not seen as prestigious a career choice as medicine indicates two problems: first, that care-giving and nurturing, a central (though certainly not the only) function of professional nursing is not seen as important or essential. The second problem involves the difficulty in recruiting people, men or women, to a profession that is devalued and misunderstood.

This devalued image of the nurse results from long-held and unattractive stereotypes as well as a misunderstanding of what it is they actually do. It is often hard for the public to know how to identify a nurse among other healthcare personnel. In "The Image of Nursing: Past, Present and Future," (*Imprint,* February/March 2002, *www.nsna.org*), Michael Evans, a member of the Board of Directors of NSNA and editor of *Imprint*, its official publication, writes that there is a disconnect on the part of the public about nurses. One problem is the representation of the nurse in the media which shows "her" in a white uniform and cap, both of which were discarded by nurses in the late '70s and early '80s in favor of the more relaxed look of colorful scrubs. While the scrubs are the preferred garb today, they can create confusion in determining who the professional nurse caregiver is among the myriad of healthcare personnel who all dress alike.[6]

Compounding the problem of the nurse's image is that the voice of the nurse is strikingly absent from the media as an expert spokesperson. "The Woodhull Study on Nursing and the Media," an oft-quoted research project conducted in 1997 by Sigma Theta Tau International (*nursingsociety.org*), published key findings, three of which are described below. (See the back of this book for information about accessing the entire study, including its important recommendations.)

- On average, nurses were cited only 3 percent of the time in hundreds of health-related articles culled from 16 major news publications.
- In seven newspapers surveyed, nurses and nursing were referenced in only four percent of the healthcare articles examined. The few references to nurses or nursing were mostly in passing.
- Articles examined during the study referred to both physicians and healthcare academics as doctors. No example was found where a nurse with a doctorate was referred to as doctor.[7]

The idea that what nurses do is dictated by and supervised by physicians is inaccurate, but firmly believed and widely pervasive. Nor is nursing usually a stepping-stone to becoming a physician, as so many people think. Nursing and medicine are collaborative professions, often sharing responsibility for the same patient, but with a different, albeit overlapping focus. Nurses are experts in wellness and coping, rather than extensions of the medical profession.

The widely used phrase *doctor's orders* refers to medical regimens that are prescribed for a patient and expected to be executed by the nurse, based on the nurse's professional judgment. Nurses who blindly carry out medical regimens without regard for how the status of the patient may indicate otherwise or the appropriateness of the order are failing in their responsibility to protect the patient from harm. Such lack of action regarding professional nursing judgment can result in discipline or revocation of one's license. The interdependence and thoughtful collaboration of the professions of nursing and medicine is usually misunderstood by the public.

EXPERIENCES OF MEN IN NURSING

Listen to the good, the bad, and the hopeful experiences of the following men who describe what it's like for them to be a nurse. In these passages you will hear examples of the barriers and obstacles described in the previous pages. Listen also for what these men have done to overcome what they were facing, as well as what still awaits to be done.

Michael Williams continues, in "President's Notes: A Journey of Rediscovery—So How Does It Feel to You?," that "Nursing continues to be a profession that allows situations to occur, like these from my own experience:

- 'Don't let yourself be promoted too soon,' I was advised. 'Hospitals have a habit of promoting men who aren't qualified.' Even today I'm haunted by the possibility that some of my promotions have been because of my gender, not my competence.

- A week before I accepted a faculty position, the men's restroom became a storage room. 'There are no men in nursing,' I was told.

- The lone male student in a class struggled to develop his physical assessment skills because he couldn't practice on female classmates, though they could practice on him.

- Recently, when a group of us were introduced as 'the critical care nurse group,' the introducer failed to acknowledge me, because he didn't see me as a nurse."

Williams goes on to say, "Admittedly, these unfortunate examples do not tell the entire story. Fortunately, I also know about experiences like these:

- The clinical instructor contacted the student to ask him, 'Do you have any questions or concerns that I could help you clarify before you start your women's health rotation?'

- 'I need a nurse to assist me,' the obstetrician told the delivery room nurse manager, who responded, 'Let me introduce you to your patient's nurse, he is right here.'

- 'Your [female] classmates seem to have a problem that my nurse is a man,' the 19-year-old woman said to the male student. 'I don't see anything unusual about a man being a nurse, do you?'

- When the new graduate was asked why she chose nursing as a career, she replied, 'Because my father is a nurse.'"

Don Paradise is a nursing student at Mount Saint Mary's College in Newburgh, NY. In an article called "Paradise Lost No More," by Alan Snel (*Advance For Nurses*, June 24, 2002, *nursing.advanceweb.com/main.aspx*), Paradise is described as "emblematic of the new face of nurses." He is a 25-year-old, six-foot-six-inch senior who played for his college's basketball team and one day wants to be an emergency flight nurse. While completing his studies, he is working in a Level II trauma center, excited about the fast-paced action and how he is able to apply the assessment skills he's learning in school. Snel describes that Paradise:

". . . joked about how banter among female nurses dies down when he enters a room. He theorized that men might not enter nursing because they look at nursing as a feminine role. . . . 'there's no feminine side to nursing . . . I want to see men be completely comfortable in this role and not feel scrutinized.'"

The article ends with the following words of advice from Paradise: "You should do stuff to be happy. I don't think gender should have anything to do with it. You have to want to care for people."[8]

In "Still Not Much of a Guy Thing," in *Hopkins Nurse* (a publication of the Johns Hopkins Hospital), Anne Bennett Swingle profiles a number of men whose self-reported invigorating experiences being a nurse represent a turning tide. They have the following to say:

> **Tom Galloway**, a veteran emergency medicine nurse says that, "Nearly one quarter of all R.N.s in emergency medicine are men, and that's enough to turn the traditional equations upside down." According to Swingle, "Galloway recalls shifts in the ER when all the doctors were women and all the nurses were men."
>
> The first job for **Kevin McDonald**, a new B.S.N. graduate, was in the cardiac surgical ICU. "It's quite a trip," McDonald says, looking back on all he learned. "The acuity of the patients is high; you really have to have the stomach for it." He goes on to say, "I have friends who make more money, but when I compare my average day to theirs, mine is more challenging and exciting. And when I describe the sort of things I do every day, they are awestruck."
>
> **Chris Boyle**, who has been a psychiatric nurse for 15 years, has been able to find all the variety and satisfaction he's ever needed without ever leaving the floor. "At every point, whenever I wanted something new, an opportunity would always open up." This included participating in opening up a day hospital where he is now the nurse manager, supervising a staff of 45 R.N.'s and other caregivers.
>
> A long time psychiatric nurse, **Gary Dunn** leads a monthly support group for male students at the Hopkins School of Nursing. Dunn started the group when he became aware that the students missed having a peer group and role models. A common problem with which they often struggle is that their family and friends see nursing as a stepping-stone to becoming a physician.[9]

NURSING'S FUTURE AND NURSING'S ROOTS

In nursing, we are living in an era between a profession dominated by women and one that is gender-neutral; a time that foretells that the term *male nurse* will fade from use, replaced by the word *nurse* to describe both men and women who perform that role. In many ways this change to gender-neutrality will reconnect nursing with its ancient and not so distant historical roots, well documented in the award-winning website "Men in American Nursing History" by Bruce Wilson, R.N., Ph.D.

(*www.geocities.com/~brucewilson*). Read what Wilson has to say and recognize how the sure-to-be increase of men in nursing is about to circle us back to our roots:

"Since the earliest times, men and women have been engaged in the practices we today call nursing. These individuals combined biological, nutritional, social, aesthetic, and spiritual support. While they have been called medicine men or witch doctors, these terms indicate a lack of understanding of the significance of their contribution, and that the healer may have been either gender.

The first nursing school in the world was started in India in about 250 BC. Only men were considered 'pure' enough to become nurses.

In the New Testament, the Good Samaritan paid the innkeeper to provide care for an injured man. No one thought it odd that a man should be paid to provide nursing care.

In every plague that swept Europe, men risked their lives to provide nursing care. A group of men, the Parabolani, in 300 AD started a hospital and provided nursing care during the black plague epidemic.

Seventy years before the Pilgrims landed on Plymouth Rock, Fray (Friar) Juan de Mena was shipwrecked off the south Texas coast. He is the first identified nurse in what was to become the United States.

During the Civil War, both sides had military men serving as nurses although we only hear about the Union volunteers, who were predominately female. The Confederate Army identified thirty men per regiment to care for the wounded. Men, including the poet, Walt Whitman, served as volunteers in the Union Army. Whitman's actual "Hospital Note Book" in his own handwriting can be viewed at *shorl.com/hufrymedepravu* and provides not only an amazing glimpse into the Civil War experience, but, perhaps for many nurses, a missing link to our history as well.

OPENING THE GLASS GATE: HOW TO ATTRACT MEN INTO THE NURSING PROFESSION

The conditions, myths, and stereotypes that inhibited free access to and equal opportunity within the nursing profession for men and women alike in the 20th century can not and must not continue into the 21st century. Recognizing that barriers

119

must be identified and removed, many individuals, organizations, and institutions are developing strategies for recruiting and retaining male nurses. Everyone within the healthcare industry, most especially nurses, needs to take responsibility for the part they play in constructing, maintaining, and ultimately eliminating the Glass Gate.

Healthcare Organizations

"Nurses for a Healthier Tomorrow" is a coalition of 37 nursing and healthcare organizations (*nursesource.org*) working together to launch an extensive communications and advertising campaign, which they describe as a grassroots effort aimed at increasing the attractiveness of nursing as a profession. Their print advertisements and public service announcements present an image of nursing as a career for everyone, inclusive of all minorities, including men, in which professionalism, teamwork, and leadership are key. The theme, *"Nursing, It's Real. It's Life."* accompanies the ads that have been shown in movie theatres and on television, and on full-color posters with pictures and career profiles of men in nursing featured prominently.[10]

Johnson & Johnson™, the world's most comprehensive manufacturer of healthcare products, has launched "The Campaign for Nursing's Future," a multiyear, national initiative to celebrate nurses and their contributions, as well as to recruit them and the faculty to train them. This highly acclaimed effort, which was developed in collaboration with nursing organizations, schools, hospitals, and other healthcare groups, and will be sustained with the assistance of an advisory group of nursing leaders, features men prominently in their print and television ads, titled, "Because I'm a Nurse" and "Dare to Care." Their website (*discovernursing.com*) features career information and dozens of profiles of male and female R.N.s and nursing students.

The broadening of diversity among healthcare workers by including men as well as other underutilized personnel sources is among the recommendations of the American Hospital Association (AHA) for solving the crisis of the nursing shortage (AHA Commission on Workforce for Hospitals and Health Systems, entitled *In Our Hands: How Hospital Leaders Can Build a Thriving Workforce, aha.org*) The Commission identified five keys to solving its workforce shortages and has charged its membership with implementing them. One of these five keys is to broaden the base of its workers by:

- Aggressively developing a more diverse workforce pool
- Creating attraction strategies for each generational cohort

- Pursuing people from the full range of potential sources
- Communicating a positive, satisfying, and inspiring image of healthcare careers

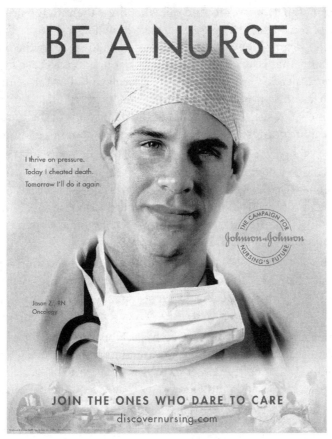

Source: Johnson & Johnson, The Campaign for Nursing's Future[11]

Colleges and Schools of Nursing

In their *Issue Bulletin*, "Effective Strategies for Increasing Diversity in Nursing Programs," the American Association of Colleges in Nursing (*www.aacn.nche.edu*)

examines some of the techniques that are working to recruit men and minorities that can be duplicated across the country. These are described below.

- The University of Texas Health Science Center at Houston convened a forum of male nurses to find out what drew them to the profession. Some of the advice they gave as described by Patricia Stark, D.S.N., R.N., F.A.A.N., dean of the School of Nursing, was to "play up the macho aspects of nursing, that is, emergency care and trauma, to advertise for students in the sports pages, and play up the longhorn symbol of UT. And, they told us to go back and proof our recruitment brochures and take out any flowery, feminine language." This resulted in the percentage of male students jumping to an impressive 29 percent of the student population.

- As part of a gift of $1.2 million given to The University of Maryland from Gilden Integrated™, a Baltimore-based public relations firm, a comprehensive marketing campaign was developed to focus on the many career opportunities in nursing. An ethnically diverse mix of men and women was featured which is credited, in part, for a 37-percent increase in applications in the fall of 2001.

- Nancy Mills, Ph.D., R.N., dean at the University of Missouri—Kansas City School of Nursing, used a federal grant to launch a three-year project to increase enrollment, specifically targeting men and minority groups and resulting in a class composed of 15 percent men.

- Mount Carmel College of Nursing has established the Learning Trails program that provides one-on-one attention and mentoring to assist men throughout their college experience. This program has helped the school achieve retention and graduation rates that exceed the national average.

- In the 2001–2002 academic year, the efforts of The College of Nursing at the University of Nebraska Medical Center to reach out to men and minorities were rewarded by an increase in the applications and admissions of male students to 54 percent and 77 percent respectively. Among the strategies used were updating the marketing materials to include images and colors that were "male-friendly."

Doing Your Part to Open the Glass Gate

Described in the passage that follows are recruitment strategies suggested by Michael Williams. Listen to his voice; select at least one idea and do it. Encourage others to do so as well. Spread the word. Practice proactivity. Participate in eliminating the Glass Gate!

"So, how will we overcome these challenges? Certainly not alone. We will need the understanding of not only our professional colleagues, but also others who are influential in changing traditional thinking. I say:

To all nurses: Speak with young people and community organizations about health careers. Socialize them to think of nursing as a career for women and men alike.

To men who are nurses: Make mentoring an essential ingredient of your professional work. If you're experienced, include men among your mentees. If you're a novice, include men among your mentors. Consider participating in career days at middle and high schools, as well as community youth groups. Make yourself visible to overcome invisibility!

To women who are nurses: Work with men in nursing to model effective communication across genders. Give us directions, even when we may forget to ask for them! Don't relegate them to [lifting] the obese patients because they have more strength. And don't assume nursing salaries will go up simply because there are more men in the profession. It's the work that matters, not the gender of the provider!

To parents and guidance counselors: When a boy who is caring, compassionate, intelligent, and adept in science is considering a health-related career, be sure that nursing is among the very real possibilities they consider.

To those developing solutions to the nursing shortage: Include men in promotional materials and develop recruitment initiatives aimed at men.

To outplacement consultants: Highlight nursing as a profession for both men and women.

To deans of nursing: Strive for greater gender diversity within the faculty. Highlight nursing faculty who are men, encouraging them to include male students among their mentees.

To managers: Instead of questioning the qualifications of male nurses who are promoted and anticipating their mistakes, encourage them. Coach them and mold them to be great leaders. Stop speculating that men are promoted only because they are men. Instead, assume that these men are expert and caring clinicians.

To philanthropists: Support nursing scholarship programs for underrepresented groups that include men among them.

And to patients and families: Whenever you encounter a health professional whose role is unknown, ask the person, 'Are you a nurse?'

As our professional journey continues, I foresee a place and time when the media reports about redistribution of gender demographics within traditional men's professions will be accompanied by articles that feature the growing redistribution of gender demographics within nursing as a traditional women's profession.

So, how does it feel? Sometimes different, other times normal, but mostly, my journey with you, it feels good!

This is how I see it. How about you?"

THE OTHER SIDE OF THE GLASS GATE

Just as women changed and are changing the face of medicine, so will men (and other minorities) change the face of nursing, with benefits occurring for nurses, physicians, and ultimately the patients they care for. Because men and women are different, the presence of more men is quite likely to influence nursing's relationship styles and communication patterns, particularly with physicians, which historically have been troubled and problematic.

That men and women are different is captured in the phrase "men are from Mars and women are from Venus," the title of a best-selling book that describes how the styles of relating, patterns of communicating, attributes, and viewpoints of each gender naturally create differences, and how despite them, both men and women benefit and learn from one another.

Alternatively, when men or women are the dominant gender in a group, there is the potential for the extremes of stereotypical feminine and masculine attributes to develop. A developmental goal of each individual, male or female, is to work toward wholeness, one characteristic of which is the capacity to embrace and express both the masculine and feminine characteristics that naturally exist within them. This developmental task is often hampered by certain cultural influences and teachings such as "little boys don't cry" and "little girls can't be angry." The gender-dominated professions of nursing and medicine, with their styles of relating and communicating frequently based on the feminine and masculine extremes described in the next chart, make the capacity for achieving balance challenging for both nurses and physicians.

The Masculine-Feminine Continuum

Potential Masculine Characteristics	Balanced Masculine and Feminine	Potential Feminine Characteristics
Anger	Emotional stability	Depression
Arrogance	Equality	Inferiority
Avoids showing vulnerability	Flexible	Avoids showing strength
Blaming	Learns from mistakes	Excusing
Ordering	Listening	Pleading
Denies feelings	In touch with feelings	Hysterical
Domineering	Creative	Victimized
Know-it-all	Curious	Knows nothing

Balance is a characteristic of the 21st-century nurse, whether male and female. As Michael Williams concludes: "Nevertheless, I am convinced that bringing male and female perspectives equally to the point of care will enrich our profession and benefit our patients and families."

MEN + WOMEN AS NURSES = BALANCE

The fact that so few men are nurses has contributed to an interpersonal environment within the profession in which a nonassertive "feminine" extreme often represents its collective behavior, as documented in the professional literature. While there are outstanding exceptions to this among individuals and nursing groups, there is yet to be heard the proactive and unified voice of clarity and authority, of which nurses are quite capable, but is more typical of other professions, most notably, medicine.

The men in the female nurse's professional life are usually not other nurses, but rather, physicians and administrators, who occupy positions of authority and power. While women also occupy these positions, they are fewer in number. It is an unfortunate reality that rather than working collaboratively, the nursing and medical professions frequently work hierarchically. The physician is in the dominant role, frequently expressing the behaviors characteristic of the masculine extremes noted in the chart on the preceding page, while the nurse typically is implicitly expected to behave in ways more closely aligned with characteristics representative of the feminine extreme. This has been and continues to be a major source of conflict for nurses that contributes to stressful work environments. It would be hard to find a nurse who hasn't had a first-hand experience and/or been witness to a physician's disruptive behavior, oft times aimed at a nurse, and rarely dealt with effectively, if at all, by administrators.

Alan H. Rosenstein, M.D., M.B.A., the physician-author of an important study titled "Nurse-Physician Relationships: Impact on Nurse Satisfaction and Retention," published in the *American Journal of Nursing*, the official publication of the American Nurses Association (*nursingcenter.com,* June 2002), corroborates this. The study (which began in July 2001 and is ongoing) surveyed nurses about their experience with and perceptions of the physicians they worked with. It concluded that disruptive physician behavior and the institutional response to it do indeed affect nurses' morale.

Rosenstein verifies that ". . . some of the issues of concern to nurses are deeply entrenched in the male-dominated physician and administrative cultures of hospitals, in which nursing is viewed as a subservient role and disruptive physician behavior is tolerated."[12] In an editorial that discusses the study, Diana Mason, the editor-in-chief of the *American Journal of Nursing* (Editorial, June 2002, *nursingworld.org/ajn*), called the nurse-physician relationships a "tired old dance, mired in gender inequity and historic precedent. She called the survey's physician-author "courageous" for disseminating it and called on nurses to take responsibility for their role in perpetuating it by "changing their own steps."[13] One way, among many, that the power structure in healthcare might be influenced and equalized is by an increase in the number of men in nursing and women in medicine.

THE WOUND DRESSER

Walt Whitman's perceptions of the sufferings of the men he cared for as a nurse as well as his efforts on their behalf are described in his moving poem, "The Dresser." Read these sections from the poem and allow them to shatter what Michael Williams called "the most devaluing [myth] of all, the perception that a man cannot be caring and compassionate enough to be a nurse."

The Wound Dresser

Bearing the bandages, water and sponge,
Straight and swift to my wounded I go,
Where they lie on the ground after the battle brought in,
Where their priceless blood reddens the grass, the ground,
Or, to the rows of the hospital tent, or under the roof's hospital,
To the long rows of cots up and down each side I return,
To each and all one after another I draw near, not one do I miss,
An attendant follows holding a tray, he carries a refuse pail,
Soon to be filled with clotted rags and blood, emptied, and fill'd again.

I onward go, I stop,
With hinged knees and steady hand to dress wounds,
I am firm with each, the pangs are sharp yet avoidable,
One turns to me his appealing eyes—poor boy! I never knew you,
Yet I think I could not refuse this moment to die for you, if that would save you.

On, on I go (open doors of time! Open hospital doors!)
The crush'd head I dress, (poor crazed hand tear not the bandage away,)
The neck of the cavalry-man with the bullet through and through I examine,
Hard the breathing rattles, quite glazed already the eye, yet life struggles hard,
(Come sweet death! Be persuaded O beautiful death! In mercy come quickly!)

From the stump of the arm, the amputated hand,
I undo the clotted lint, remove the slough,
Wash off the matter and blood,
Back on his pillow the soldier bends with
Curv'd neck and side falling head,
His eyes are closed, his face is pale, he
Dares not look on the bloody stump,
And has not yet look'd on it.

—Walt Whitman[14]

PART TWO

Converting Your Nursing Career Into *You, Inc.*

CHAPTER 9

Becoming the Nurse CEO of *You, Inc.*

In 1996, at the height of the organizational restructuring and downsizing that helped shape the landscape of today's healthcare industry, William Bridges, author *of Job Shift: How to Prosper in a Workplace Without Jobs,* advocated a whole new way of looking at work and at employment. He described a paradigm shift and a way to reframe how you think about your work that is just as essential today. He advised workers everywhere to manage their careers by converting themselves into a business, and "to see yourself as a self-contained economic entity, not as a component part looking for a whole within which you can function." This shift in thinking from *having a job* to *managing your career* is just as valuable in today's healthcare environment because it fosters the empowerment and autonomy needed for professional satisfaction. To see yourself as a self-contained economic entity would mean that your mental attitude is one of self-employment whether you work for others or for yourself.

The following ways of thinking about your work expand on Bridges's advice:

- Be "vendor-minded." In nursing practice, this would translate into being "consumer-oriented," recognizing that everyone, the patient, your coworkers, your employer, and, of course, yourself, are consumers.

- See yourself surrounded by a marketplace, with limitless options, whether or not you are on the payroll of an organization.

- Join, rather than blindly work for, your organization and customers (patients).

- Think like an entrepreneur, or in the case of the employed nurse, an "intrapreneur," by identifying or creating new work opportunities.

- Be independent as well as interdependent, relying on yourself as well as collaborating with others.
- Find new and creative ways to contribute your skills and competencies in current and emerging healthcare marketplaces.
- Commit to continuous learning.
- Create meaningful work, believing in the contribution you have to make.[1]

Bridges was not a lone voice in this seemingly unconventional world of reframing how we were thinking about jobs and work at that time. In 1996, *U.S. News and World Report,* a very conventional, mainstream publication, devoted 32 pages to an article entitled, *"You, Inc."* The article described how all United States industries, including healthcare:

> ". . . have leapt headlong into the information age, and how careers will never again be the same . . . At no time in modern history have so many workers been so totally reliant on their own wits and resources to thrive . . . the upshot: 'You, Inc.' may be the fastest growing employment segment in the economy, as people learn to invest in themselves as if they were a corporation."[2]

Invest in yourself as if you were a corporation! What an empowering phrase! What would *your* work, *your* life look like if you were to take this phrase and seriously apply it to your nursing career, if you considered yourself as the chief executive officer (CEO) of *You, Inc.?* And likewise, how would *not* investing in all aspects of your nursing *"business,"* with the seriousness of a CEO, affect your career mobility and your professional satisfaction?

While it is true that in just a few short years we've moved from a seller's market (nursing surplus) to a buyer's market (nursing shortage), applying the concept of *You, Inc.* to your nursing career is as relevant and timely as ever. Utilizing the principles of *You, Inc.* can help you shape your career path, ensuring that you can take advantage of exciting, new work options as they emerge, as well as deepen your professional satisfaction with the work you may be currently doing.

The Nurse CEO of *You, Inc.*

Professional Experience

- Possesses targeted, progressive, cumulative work experience as a generalist and/or a specialist
- Can articulate examples of work experiences that have added value to the workplace
- Is aware of, able to support, and can contribute to patient-focused care in a consumer-oriented business environment
- Knows his/her transferable skills
- Is cross-trained
- Seeks continuing education
- Is computer literate and Internet savvy
- Earns the Bachelor of Science in Nursing
- Pursues advanced educational preparation commensurate with career goals
- Receives ANCC board-certification as a generalist, specialist, or other professional certification
- Seeks professional memberships

Personal Characteristics

- Is flexible, adaptive, assertive, confident, empowered
- Is self-directed and team-oriented
- Strives to be an innovative problem solver
- Does not accept the status quo
- Is willing to take risks
- Learns from mistakes
- Resolves conflicts
- Thinks critically
- Is a master networker

A primary mission of *You, Inc.* is the continuous exploration of the following questions:

- How are the skills and competencies you have to offer (your nursing "business") as good or perhaps even better than that of others?
- What makes you at least as qualified, or more?
- What contributions can you or are you making to the mission of the organization where you are working, or from whom you are seeking employment?
- In what ways have you or will you improve the quality of service that the organization provides, over and above the minimum requirement of showing up for work and performing the tasks required in the job description?

These questions are important because while healthcare may be in a post-downsizing era (at least as far as professional nursing jobs are concerned), we are still operating in a managed care environment. This means that organizational viability will still be driven by the bottom line. If a particular activity (a nursing job or role, for example) cannot somehow be translated into direct or indirect profit, it cannot continue unchanged if the organization is to survive. Harsh as this may sound, this kind of thinking does not have to be mutually exclusive from caring for and about patients. More importantly, it is seen as *the way* to care, as a roadmap for providing high quality patient care, as long as it is tempered with sound ethical and moral standards. Since this is a reality in today's healthcare marketplace, it needs to be a reality for *You, Inc.* as well.

To manage and administer *You, Inc.* most effectively, you need to know the ways in which your business, your product/service, if you will, is different from that of others. You also need to be assertive enough to express these personal and professional attributes in performance appraisals, on your resume, during interviews, and so on. You should aim to get as close as you can to having the professional experiences and personal characteristics described on the next page. You should have a plan for developing those attributes you don't yet have, seeing yourself as a work in progress, evolving towards the same kind of continuous quality improvement as the healthcare organizations for which you may be working.

The Nurse CEO of *You, Inc.*

Organization or Corporation	*You, Inc.*
Has a mission statement, a clearly stated purpose	Has a mission statement aligned with values and a vision
Has an operating license	Has an R.N. license, and perhaps others
Insured against malpractice	Carries malpractice insurance and accidental injury claims; other insurance as indicated
Operates based on written standards of practice	Utilizes ANA Standards in the practice of nursing
Abides by ethical standards	Abides by the ANA Code of Ethics
Utilizes policies and procedures for the delivery of its services and the fulfillment of its mission	Develops policies and procedures that determine where, when, and for how long *You, Inc.* will provide its services in a particular segment of the healthcare marketplace
Engages in continuous quality improvement programs	Engages in continuous training and education to improve the quality and marketability of skills and services
Seeks and applies for recognition by associations and accrediting agencies for outstanding achievement and excellence in service, such as Magnet Hospital Status awarded by ANCC	Seeks out recognition for professional achievement through ANCC board certification, or through other professional associations. Uses Magnet Hospital Status as one criterion for choosing employment
Builds alliances, coalitions, networks, and partnerships with other organizations	Considers itself a partner to healthcare organizations, the organization has patients that need healthcare services; *You, Inc.* provides those services and builds professional and personal networks
Competes effectively with other organizations that provide the same service by means of effective marketing and public relations	Adapts business strategies to position *You, Inc;* utilizes business strategies to compete effectively, including product development, market research, advertising (resume), sales (interviewing), networking strategies, and the development of a marketing plan

135

As you compare the two lists, you may recognize that most of the expectations and functions necessary for *You, Inc.* aren't too different from what is expected of nurses who want career excellence, except perhaps for the last item about utilizing business strategies as a career management tool. To make this shift, imagine yourself as the Chief Executive Officer (CEO) of *You, Inc.*, situated in some central place in your home, your own "Nursing Office," if you will, your own headquarters of operation. From this place you can plan, implement, and track the activities of *You, Inc.*, as well as oversee and coordinate the departments of *You, Inc.* listed below.

The Nurse CEO of *You, Inc.*

You, Inc.	Department Responsibilities and Functions
Product Development	In charge of developing and articulating who you are and what you have to offer, including your mission statement, values and needs, vision, and preferred nursing roles and competencies
Market Research	Conducts ongoing research and makes recommendations about where along the continuum of care *You, Inc.*'s nursing skills and competencies are most needed; determines how best to take advantage of newly emerging healthcare opportunities
Advertising	Creates and revises *You, Inc.*'s resume and maintains a professional portfolio
Sales	Develops and hones techniques for interviewing in order to "sell" *You, Inc.*'s nursing skills and competencies most effectively
Networking	Creates and maintains professional and personal alliances and relationships
Marketing Plan	Performs ongoing assessments of needs and develops strategic career plans with defined goals, stated tasks, and specific timelines

PROFILE OF A NURSE CEO OF *YOU, INC.*

Debbie, a single parent of a two-year-old daughter, demonstrates how *You, Inc.* can work. She is a fee-for-service (per diem) home-care nurse who works for several home-care agencies simultaneously. She pays for her own and her daughter's health and disability insurance and has recently established a private retirement fund managed by a financial adviser at her local bank.

She is an ANCC-certified, medical-surgical nurse practicing at the generalist level and will soon complete an adult nurse practitioner program paid for by scholarships, savings targeted for starting school, and one low-interest loan. The work she does at the home care agency is aligned with her work values of autonomy and independence, and supports *You, Inc.'s* mission of influencing the physical and emotional health of older adults. Her long-term vision is to create more in-home mental health services, especially for the isolated home-bound patients that make up the majority of her practice and for whom very little mobile support is available.

Debbie arranges her work schedule and maintains an adequate income so that it best supports her school goals and parenting responsibilities by reducing the number of hours she is available to the agencies when school is in session, and increasing them during semester breaks. She is careful about the kind of assignments she accepts when she is in school, choosing lighter assignments such as home health aide supervisions, which require less of a long-term commitment than carrying her own caseload of patients. Debbie self-manages the components of work life traditionally managed by employers, including health and disability insurance, retirement savings, tuition reimbursement, time scheduling, and patient assignments. She carries her own malpractice insurance. She misses the natural relationship-building that goes on in workplaces where people are in the same building all day, but substitutes school-based involvement when classes are in session and tries to attend professional meetings during semester breaks.

EMPOWERMENT

In some ways, the influence of managed care really created two revolutions in healthcare. One revolution was about the structure of the industry itself, and the other was about the shift in the thinking and behavior of the people in it. Both revolutions will continue to influence the nursing profession in the 21st century.

While the downsizing of professional nursing jobs has ended, role restructuring and the cost-containment influence of managed care has not. Healthcare systems will continue to restructure and reorganize themselves to reduce costs. An example of restructuring that could easily affect you is the merger of two medical centers. Suppose you were a nurse on an inpatient pediatric unit in a large metropolitan medical center that has just merged with another, which also has a full service pediatric center. An initial response as the CEO of *You, Inc.* should be to conduct marketplace research in order to determine what pediatric services are now being duplicated and what will possibly be reorganized as a result of this new affiliation. This will begin to give you the information you need to determine how best to position yourself in this new environment, or if you even want to, knowing now that roles and responsibilities are likely to change.

Being the CEO of *You, Inc.* means recognizing that while the *employer* owns the job you do, *you* are the one who owns the work that is being done! Developing this kind of thinking about your work empowers you to assume more responsibility for the shape and direction your work will take. And, this will ultimately influence your fulfillment with your nursing career.

The Unspoken Employment Contract

The unspoken contract between employer and employee that has existed since the Industrial Revolution has been traditionally responsible for determining the quality and longevity of the employment relationship, while encouraging over-reliance on the direction of others, and limiting the degree of personal empowerment. Influenced by the new understanding that today's complex workplace requires mutuality and collaboration, rather than the hierarchical decision-making of the past, a new employment contract is emerging, with employers expecting a much more empowered employee. This shift in thinking, which has important implications for nursing career planning, is well-described by David Noer in *Healing the Wounds* in the following comparison:

Old Employment Contract

- Tenure and long-term relationships
- Linear promotion as reward for performance, within fixed job descriptions
- Lifetime employment through loyalty to the organization, which provides long-term career paths and discourages external hiring

This approach resulted in a workforce that was older, nondiverse, plateaued, demotivated, codependent, and mediocre; the potential for empowerment was limited.

New Employment Contract

- Employment is situational with flexible, portable benefit plans
- Blurred distinction between full-time, part-time, and temporary employees
- Reward for performance is based on tenure-free acknowledgement of contribution achieved through self-directed work teams and nonhierarchical performance systems
- Employees are more autonomous
- Loyalty means responsibility and good work within nontraditional career paths[3]

This approach can result in a mobile workforce that is flexible, motivated, task-invested, empowered, and responsible.

The Empowerment Continuum

To be empowered is to act on your own behalf. To be empowered is to refuse to be trapped without options, *no matter what!* Empowerment means staying loyal to yourself, your needs and values, your professional and personal mission and vision, all the while committing yourself to the goals of the organization for the time you are there. It is remembering that your *work* is portable: it belongs to you, and that what belongs to the organization is the *job* you are occupying for awhile. Empowerment is the essence of the self-employed attitude; it is what fuels the Nurse CEO of *You, Inc.*

Empowerment can be envisioned as existing on a continuum, moving from the least empowered to the most empowered behaviors, from an employee mentality to a self-employed attitude (see box on next page). As you might imagine, the most empowered behaviors correlate with a self-employed attitude.

The Empowerment Continuum can be a useful professional growth tool, serving as a guide to your professional development, as well as a way to benchmark or measure your success. We will revisit the concept of empowerment in the chapter on "The Resilient Nurse." During this nursing shortage when nurses are being asked to do so much more with fewer resources, empowerment, the capacity to act on your own behalf, to say no to unreasonable requests, and to advocate for your own well-being *as well as* safe nursing care standards has never been more important.

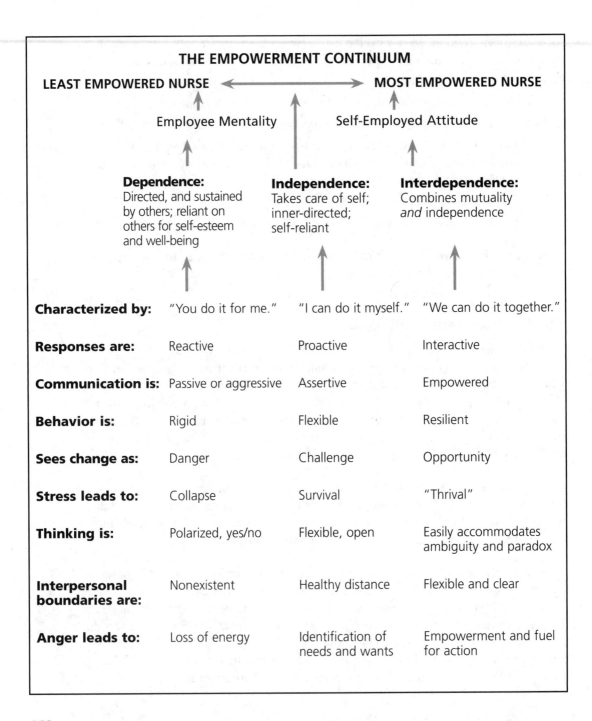

THE EMPOWERMENT CONTINUUM

LEAST EMPOWERED NURSE ⟵⟶ MOST EMPOWERED NURSE

Employee Mentality   Self-Employed Attitude

Dependence: Directed, and sustained by others; reliant on others for self-esteem and well-being

Independence: Takes care of self; inner-directed; self-reliant

Interdependence: Combines mutuality *and* independence

Characterized by:	"You do it for me."	"I can do it myself."	"We can do it together."
Responses are:	Reactive	Proactive	Interactive
Communication is:	Passive or aggressive	Assertive	Empowered
Behavior is:	Rigid	Flexible	Resilient
Sees change as:	Danger	Challenge	Opportunity
Stress leads to:	Collapse	Survival	"Thrival"
Thinking is:	Polarized, yes/no	Flexible, open	Easily accommodates ambiguity and paradox
Interpersonal boundaries are:	Nonexistent	Healthy distance	Flexible and clear
Anger leads to:	Loss of energy	Identification of needs and wants	Empowerment and fuel for action

TOWARD A SELF-EMPLOYED ATTITUDE

To develop a self-employed attitude, several shifts in your thinking are necessary:

1. Reconceptualize the manner in which you work and where it falls on the "Continuum of Work" (see diagram below).

2. Recognize that the employer owns the job you do, while you own your very portable work and ever-expanding transferable skills.

3. Aim for empowered mutuality and interdependence in your work relationships, instead of allowing yourself to be passively dependent or overreliant on the direction of others.

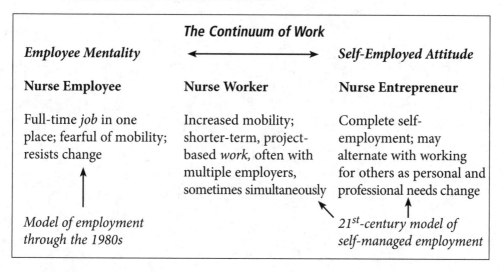

The Continuum of Work

Employee Mentality ⟷ *Self-Employed Attitude*

Nurse Employee

Full-time *job* in one place; fearful of mobility; resists change

Model of employment through the 1980s

Nurse Worker

Increased mobility; shorter-term, project-based *work,* often with multiple employers, sometimes simultaneously

Nurse Entrepreneur

Complete self-employment; may alternate with working for others as personal and professional needs change

21st-century model of self-managed employment

CHAPTER 10

The Product Development Department of *You, Inc.*

You have a product to offer others, to sell, if you will. Your nursing skills and competencies, your experience, and your transferable skills comprise your product in the form of a service that benefits others and which healthcare organizations desire to utilize for altruistic reasons as well as for profit. When you consider your product/service in this way, you establish within you a department called *You, Inc.* that shapes and directs your professional growth.

UNDERSTANDING AND STRENGTHENING *YOU, INC.*

For your product/service to be most attractive to the healthcare establishments of your choice, for your own professional satisfaction, as well as for burnout protection, two kinds of attention to your product are required: professional development and personal development. Chapter 16, "The Resilient Nurse: Self-Care Strategies," will provide you with an opportunity to explore your personal development. This chapter will give you ideas on how to strengthen your professional development.

The state of rapid change and permanent transition that characterized the downsizing era of the 1990s is the new status quo in these early years of the 21st century. Expect the areas of your professional and personal life to be fluid, to change unexpectedly, and to require fast adaptation on your part. Recognizing this will allow you to position *You, Inc.* to take best advantage of opportunities as the healthcare marketplace continues to shift.

When a change happens that affects your current job responsibilities, you have two options. The first is to realign your product by updating it to the skills now required. The second is to offer your product where it is still needed. For example, suppose you are an OR nurse in a hospital that merged with another from across town and will now be doing surgery only at that location. This newly formed medical center now finds itself with far many OR nurses and has offered you a transfer to the Cardiac Cath Lab, which will be expanding to accommodate more patients. You could choose to remain an OR nurse and offer your product/service to another employer, or you could choose to use this as an opportunity to add cardiac cath skills to your product/service.

It is possible that a marketplace shift significant enough to affect your life could occur about every six months. This change could represent a shift in healthcare itself or a shift in society, which in turn has influenced the healthcare industry. To keep current and stay aligned with changes that will occur in your work or personal life, you need to conduct periodic, perhaps biannual assessments of the current state and marketability of your product/service. Reflecting on the answers to the three questions below, as well as recognizing that the answers are sure to change over time, will insure optimal mobility and career satisfaction:

- Who are you?
- What do you have to offer?
- Who needs it?

In this chapter we will explore the answers to the first two questions. The third question will be discussed in Chapter 11, "The Market Research Department of *You, Inc.*"

WHO ARE YOU?

You are unique, you are complex; your needs and preferences may be similar to others, but how you blend those needs represents how you are different from others. Who you are as a nurse is certainly more than the job you do. Which of the following descriptions most closely resemble how you think about your nursing practice?

Job: Belongs to someone else (called the employer); is given to you for a period of time, the length of which is not necessarily determined by you; can be modified at the will of the employer, not always with your input or permission

> **Career:** A proactive experience of choice based on your life purpose (mission), guided by your vision, and grounded in your values; frequently expressed in a series of temporary work experiences called jobs[1]

The resilient, proactive, and empowered Nurse CEO of *You, Inc.* always thinks career, not job! How about you?

Your job represents your current focus within an ever-evolving career containing very portable work. Your work reflects your mission (your purpose in life), which is rooted in the values you believe in, and the vision you have for how all this fits together. Throughout your nursing career, as you periodically reflect on and refine the answers to the questions, *Who are you?* and *What do you have to offer?*, you solidify what is permanently yours, namely, your work. Owning your work in this manner creates career satisfaction, deters burnout, and strengthens your ability to withstand the winds of change, whether in the healthcare industry or elsewhere in your life.

Career Satisfaction Tree

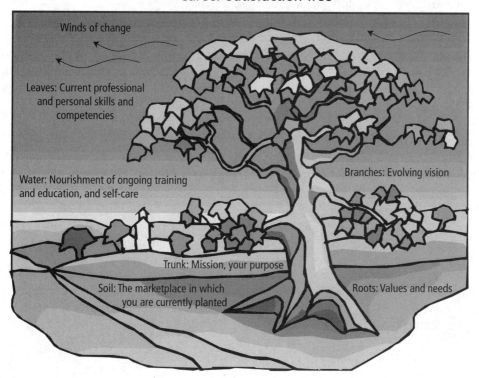

YOUR MISSION

An ad for a major New York medical center read as follows: "Providing compassionate quality healthcare isn't our job . . . it's our mission." Likewise, while *You, Inc.* may occupy a job slot for a particular employer for a certain length of time, it does so in order to enact its mission, which hopefully is aligned with that of the employer.

Developing Your Mission

A mission is the evolving expression of what you believe your life purpose to be. It is based on innate as well as learned abilities. It includes preferences for life activities (of which work is only one part) that are rooted in your value system and aligned with your vision. In her book, *The Path*, Laurie Beth Jones describes a mission statement as a:

> ". . . written-down reason for being; key to finding your path in life and to identifying the mission you choose to follow; having a clearly articulated mission statement gives one a template of purpose that can be used to initiate, evaluate, and refine all of one's activities."[2]

What is your "written-down reason for being," your "template of purpose"? Determining this is essential to forming a strong foundation upon which to build *You, Inc.* This becomes a way to keep yourself grounded even as you move forward, or a way to decide not to move in a particular direction with which your mission is not aligned.

Jones says that finding one's mission and then fulfilling it is "perhaps the most vital activity in which a person can engage." Steven Covey, author of *The Seven Habits of Highly Effective People* and *Putting First Things First*, echoes this. Covey describes a mission statement as follows:

> "A philosophy or creed which focuses on what you want to be (character) and do (contributions and achievements), and on the values (principles) upon which being and doing is based; it is a written standard, a personal constitution, and like the United States Constitution, based on self-evident truths of the Declaration of Independence; it is fundamentally changeless, defended and supported, pledged allegiance to, and enables people to ride through such major traumas as war; it empowers individuals with tireless strength in the midst of change."[3]

So many phrases in Covey's description of a mission statement have relevance to your nursing career and to *You, Inc.* For example, to pledge allegiance to yourself rather than your employer keeps you free to stay or go, depending on which way the winds of change are blowing, and most importantly, whether the change is still aligned with your mission.

In 1995, during the height of the downsizing crisis, Leah Curtin, editor of *Nursing Management*, captured the meaning of this for nurses of that time. It is still quite relevant today. She said:

> "Nurses must learn to redirect their loyalty from their employer to their work, committing themselves to self development and skills enlargement. As they invest in themselves, they become more valuable."

Where is your loyalty? To whom are you pledging allegiance? And, how is it affecting your ability to "declare" yourself "independent"? While your employer certainly warrants your *commitment* to their mission for the length of time you choose to stay, your *loyalty* and *allegiance* belongs to *You, Inc.* What "self-evident truths" are in your "personal constitution"? What will you go to "war" over, stand up for, defend, and support, no matter what? For example, in what ways might *You, Inc.* stand up for, defend, and support safe staffing ratios, adequate time for meal breaks, and the elimination of mandatory overtime?

Writing Your Mission Statement

A mission statement is not something you write overnight or in one sitting. Rather, it evolves over time. According to Covey, it takes "deep introspection, careful analysis, and thoughtful expression," as you reflect on where you've been and how it has affected you, where you want to go, and what you want your life to be about. Because it is a solid expression of your values and vision, it should not be written in isolation from them.

Jones describes the elements of a mission statement as:
- No longer than a single sentence
- Easily understood by a 12-year-old
- Able to be recited automatically, by memory
- Perfectly suited to you

In both the Covey and Jones books you will find excellent descriptions and exercises to use in developing your mission statement (see Endnotes at the back of this book). Use the following exercise, adapted from *The Path*, to get started.

There are three steps to creating your mission statement.

Step 1 = What you do, expressed in three action verbs

Step 2 = What you stand for; the principles, causes you would defend to the death; your core value or values

Step 3 = Whom you want to help; whom you really want to serve, be around, inspire, learn from, impact, and make a difference for

Step 1

Select three words from the list of action verbs below that most excite you, shed light on who you are, describe what you most like to spend your time doing. (This is a partial list based on a more complete one in *The Path*.)

facilitate	foster	alleviate	prepare	realize
communicate	improve	involve	motivate	educate
support	empower	sustain	enhance	organize

Write the three words representing what you do here: _____ _____ _____

Step 2

Write a word or key phrase that describes your core value or values, the principle or principles you would defend to the death, such as *joy* or *service* or *justice* or *independence*. For additional value words, consult the list in the Self-Assessment Exercise later on in this chapter.

Write what you stand for here: _____

Step 3

Describe those whom you want to help. The more specific, the better. Consider the kind of healthcare client, the patient population or nursing specialty, the age group, and so on.

Write whom you help here: _____

Creating Your Mission Statement

Combine the words from Steps 1, 2, and 3 to form your mission statement. Fill in the blanks below:

My mission (what I do):

_____, _____, and _____

(your three verbs from Step 1)

My values or principles (what I stand for):

_____

(your core values or principles from Step 2)

To or for, among or with (those whom you help):

_____

(the group or cause from Step 3)

Sample Mission Statement: John

John, a staff nurse in a family health clinic, wrote the following mission statement which helped him determine what his next work experience would be upon learning that the clinic had lost its grant funding and would therefore have to close:

My mission (what I do):

nurture, educate, and facilitate

My values or principles (what I stand for):

health and well-being

To or for, among or with (those whom you help):

traditional and nontraditional families, including single fathers

Having this as his mission statement helped John recognize that the employer could only take away his job, not his work, not his career, and certainly not his mission. It helped him to focus on what he wanted his next career move to be, and what employer might be most interested in what he had to offer. Within two months, he was working as a visiting nurse, making home visits to new moms and dads, many of whom were young and engaging in high-risk behaviors.

Additional examples of mission statements representative of the work nurses do include:

- Facilitate, teach, and encourage the mental and emotional health of inner-city schoolchildren.
- Inspire, recognize, and promote healing in grieving adults.
- Communicate, demonstrate, and encourage computer literacy among healthcare professionals.
- Model, nurture, and facilitate empowerment in single mothers.
- Inspire, improve, and sustain self-care and independence in "the oldest old" (people over 85).
- Develop, prepare, and circulate diabetic teaching materials for newly diagnosed children.

YOUR VALUES AND NEEDS

Values are the beliefs that ground your decisions and activities in the work world and in your personal life as well. They are the expression of deeply held beliefs about how you like things to be and what you prefer to experience. Values are often based on and influenced by psychological needs. Examples of values include: to be with people, to be independent, to be useful, to experience stability, to have influence, to serve others, and so on. See the list in the Self-Assessment Exercise for an expanded list of values.

Values shape your interests and contribute to the skills you decide to learn as well as the accomplishments you achieve. Because your values and needs form the basis for the personal interests you pursue and the career paths you select, knowing about them is essential to the question, *Who are you?*

Take Orinthia, for example, who currently works in the newborn nursery of a community hospital. She has worked in this hospital for four years and this is her third assignment in the obstetrical department, where nurses rotate for six-month periods to each clinical area, including the ambulatory care clinics. She is experiencing the same kind of boredom and restlessness that she remembers having twice before; once when she worked on the postpartum unit, and before that, when she worked in the prenatal clinic. The one time during this current rotation that she remembered feeling genuinely interested in her work was when it was decided that infants experiencing mild respiratory distress would no longer be transferred out to the neonatal intensive care unit (NICU) of a major medical center for treatment. Instead, the nurses in the newborn nursery would be taught the skills needed to care for these infants. She learned the assessment and technical skills quickly, and in fact became a resource to two of her nurse colleagues, Barbara and Joan, who found these critical care tasks overwhelming. When these nurses investigated what values and needs might be represented by their preferences for work assignments, it became clear that there were some striking differences among them. Orinthia identified the following needs and values:

Challenge—work that is mentally stimulating

Detail work—performance of tasks requiring accurate focus and attention

Fast pace—meet demanding expectations within time deadlines

Excitement—work characterized by frequent novelty and drama

Variety—frequent change in job responsibilities

Barbara and Joan, the nurses who felt overwhelmed with this new assignment, identified the following values and needs:

Predictability—satisfaction with routine, repetitious tasks

Expertise—being good at something

Mastery—acquired proficiency and expertise in tasks

Connection—giving and receiving caring, support, and warmth

While all three nurses loved working with mothers and babies, Orinthia preferred caring for the sicker infants while her peers did not. In addition, Orinthia realized that practically none of the work preferences that were representative of her values and needs were typically experienced during her past rotations to the postpartum unit or the prenatal clinic, and were only present in this current rotation to the nursery when she was assigned to care for these sick infants. During those times, she felt challenged by the potential unpredictability of the sick infant's health status and the fast-paced work requiring attention to detail that was missing for her in the routine care of well babies, exactly what her peers enjoyed.

When these nurses clarified their needs and values related to the kind of work they preferred, they were able to request work assignments that resulted in more professional satisfaction, and experienced less boredom and stress. Orinthia was assigned to care for the infants with respiratory distress whenever possible, while the other nurses performed the tasks more routinely associated with well baby care and more aligned with their values and preferences, including teaching and emotional support of new parents. Eventually, Orinthia went to work in the obstetrical department of a hospital that didn't require rotation through all the Ob-Gyn subspecialties, and was permanently assigned to the NICU, where the fast pace suited her perfectly and was aligned with her mission to *"Support, facilitate, or strengthen connection in the mother-baby bond of critically ill newborns."*

Do the exercise on the following pages to begin exploring and clarifying your needs and values as they relate to your work preferences, to your mission, to your vision, and to the larger question of *"Who are you?"* (Adapted from *The Lifetime Career Manager: New Strategies for a New Era* by James C. Cabrera and Charles F. Albrecht.)

SELF-ASSESSMENT EXERCISE: YOUR NEEDS AND VALUES

Rank the following needs and values and their descriptions according to the following scale:

1 = Always necessary. Impossible or very hard to work or live without

2 = Often necessary. Could work or live without it, if necessary, or temporarily, but wouldn't want to, would miss it a lot

3 = Sometimes necessary. Would prefer to have it, but could manage fairly well if it wasn't there

4 = Rarely or never necessary. Could easily work or live without it; don't think about it much

Score	Value	Description
_____	Achievement	Attain and maintain a sense of accomplishment and mastery
_____	Aesthetics	Work in a setting that values the beauty of things and ideas
_____	Affection	Express and receive warmth and caring
_____	Authenticity	Be genuinely yourself
_____	Balance	Achieve satisfactory proportion between work and personal life
_____	Career advancement	Experience opportunities for vertical mobility (promotion), as well as horizontal mobility (transfer) within the workplace
_____	Challenge	Experience work as mentally stimulating
_____	Competition	Achieve mastery by competing with others or by challenging yourself
_____	Creativity	Express imagination and ingenuity in work
_____	Detail work	Perform tasks requiring accurate focus and detail
_____	Efficient organization	Work in an organization that runs effectively with minimal bureaucracy

(Go on to next page.)

SELF-ASSESSMENT EXERCISE (CONT.)

_____	Excitement	Experience adventure, frequent novelty and drama
_____	Expertise	Feeling skilled, being good at something
_____	Emotional resilience	Ability to mediate and process personal feelings and bounce back from interpersonal difficulties
_____	Fast pace	Meet demanding expectations within time deadlines
_____	Family	Experience contented personal relationships or living situation
_____	Friendship	Develop social and personal relationships with peers and colleagues
_____	Health	Pursue physical, mental, and emotional well-being
_____	Helping others	Contribute to or assist others in need
_____	Independence	Control the type of work you do, including schedule
_____	Integrity	Work ethically and honestly
_____	Knowledge	Learn and use specific information
_____	Leadership	Influence, authorize, or direct others to achieve results
_____	Location	Live in a convenient geographical location in a suitable community
_____	Management	Achieve work goals as a result of the efforts of others
_____	Money	Reap significant financial rewards
_____	Meaningful work	Perform work that has purpose, relevance

(Go on to next page.)

SELF-ASSESSMENT EXERCISE (CONT.)

_____	Personal growth	Develop and grow into your potential
_____	Pleasure	Experience enjoyment, fun, satisfaction
_____	Physical health	Express vitality and well being
_____	Positive atmosphere	Work in a pleasing, supportive, harmonious setting
_____	Power	Control the resources at work
_____	Recognition	Receive credit and appreciation for work well done; be known or well-known; be praised
_____	Security	Work without fear of unemployment, have stable future
_____	Service	Contribute to the well-being, welfare, or satisfaction of another
_____	Spirituality	Express meaning of life or religious beliefs
_____	Status	Attain a position of recognized importance
_____	Variety and change	Perform tasks of great variety
_____	Wisdom	Develop insight and understanding
_____	Work with others	Belong to a satisfying work group or team

Interpreting Your Score

In reviewing this self-assessment, notice how many 1s and 2s you have and whether your work or personal life is set up to allow their expression. The 1s and 2s relate to values and needs that should not be compromised—at least not for too long, because compromising them can lead to personal and interpersonal conflict, stress, and eventually to burnout. The 3s and 4s are places where you can allow more compromise as you attempt to align *You, Inc.* with the reality of any given situation.

You may be living out of balance and harmony with who you are if your values and needs are blocked from expression. While it is unrealistic to expect the workplace to match all of your needs and values, a preponderance of them should be met for you to feel satisfied and productive. A value system that is very misaligned with the work you are doing is a perfect prescription for stress. Should you find yourself in this situation, consider the following options:

Compensate for Your Unmet Values

Compensate for missing values by identifying other places for their expression. Perhaps you could take courses, enroll in seminars, join a support group, or engage in a personal inquiry through psychotherapy.

Negotiate for Your Values

Negotiate for the value or need that is not being fulfilled. For example, if you scored a 1 or 2 for recognition, and it is in short supply where you work, try asking for feedback more often or consider participating in a work activity that might provide some consistent appreciation for a job well done, perhaps committee work.

Realign Your Values

This does not mean giving up what keeps you rooted to the essence of who you are. To realign your values means to evaluate what your current job can realistically provide and to see if you can modify your expectations accordingly. This might be possible if you know that the job you have is temporary, or if you design your personal life so that there are ample opportunities for the expression of the needs or values blocked at work.

For example, if you scored a 1 or 2 for "power" (controlling resources at work) and this is not possible within your current job responsibilities, try relating to what is there, not what you wish could be, and learn to let go of what you cannot control. This could be a growth experience for you as you learn to adjust and accommodate to the reality of your situation, rather than fighting to change the unchangeable. When you have not succeeded in changing something you don't like, and you decide to stay in the situation anyway, you will find relief from the tension this creates by changing the way you think about it. Marcel Proust captured this idea well when he said:

> "The real voyage of discovery consists not in seeking new landscapes but in having new eyes."

Where might you need to change how you think about or see something?

Keep in mind that selecting this option requires paying very careful attention to the fine line between flexibility and total compromise of one's needs and values. Many acute care nurses, and nurses in general, are faced with this dilemma because of the higher volume of sicker patients requiring care during shorter lengths of stay in these times of managed care and fiscal restraint. The phrase "do more with less" is an affront to the nursing profession's collective values regarding the provision of safe and ethical care, and individual nurses need to carefully examine what can be compromised and what cannot.

Another situation that requires some realignment of values is what you think or feel about healthcare establishments utilizing business principles and philosophies to run their organizations. Is caring for others mutually exclusive from running a business? Is it possible to have a business/bottom-line mentality and still provide compassionate and empathic care? Coming to terms with this reality requires moving away from black and white, either-or kind of thinking and finding a middle ground where the values of caring and business can coexist side by side. This kind of reframing and revisioning is necessary for complex issues like these, helping the nurse to discover the "new eyes" that Proust wrote of in the quotation above.

Honor and Stand Up for Your Values

Decide whether a career move, and perhaps a new career path, is necessary because your values are either too compromised, or just cannot be met where you are. If control of resources is essential to you and realigning your expectations is not possible, ask yourself why you're working in a place that can't meet these needs. If your answer has more to do with salary and employment benefits than your overall career goals, you might benefit from reexamining and prioritizing your needs and values with a mentor or coach who can provide objective feedback and guidance. If you believe that the latest changes in your workplace have made it impossible to provide safe, effective care, you would be better off working where your values and needs about patient care delivery could more easily be met. So would your employer, and so would the patients you care for.

Another way to stand up for what you believe in is to assist others in fighting for what you are not able to influence on your own. For example, supporting the legislative efforts of your state nurses' association as it addresses safe staffing guidelines and whistle-blower laws. Joining the American Nurses Association and participating directly through committee work or indirectly though membership dues is another way to honor and stand up for your nursing practice values.

DEVELOPING YOUR VISION

Robert Kennedy said, "Some men see things as they are and ask, 'Why?' I dream of the things that could be and ask, 'Why not?'" Kennedy had a vision of the future that he believed in. Do you? A vision of what you want for the immediate or even distant future is necessary for *You, Inc.* A vision is a place for your hopes and dreams to grow; it is a guidepost for your plans and goals; it is where your mission and your values will still make sense even though they will be shaped and refined in the process of getting there.

Having a vision of the future provides a stabilizing anchor in the present that can steady you through turbulent times, while serving as a beacon of hope and optimism toward which you navigate. A vision can become a powerful self-care and stress management strategy because it prevents you from feeling trapped or victimized in a situation that may no longer be aligned with your mission or values. A vision gives you some realistic control over your destiny, especially if you use your present experience as a training ground to accumulate the skills and experiences that will transfer to what you envision yourself doing in the future.

For example, Clarissa values teaching and enjoys helping people feel more confident in their ability to learn complicated things. She has been working as an acute care nurse on a medical unit for four years and especially likes helping newly diagnosed diabetics feel less overwhelmed as they learn to manage their own care. Because of the nursing shortage, Clarissa has found herself with additional work assignments that allow her less time for teaching, even though this is still an expected part of her job. In taking stock of her present situation as well as what she envisions herself doing in the future, she imagines combining her nursing knowledge and the knack she has for teaching complicated concepts in a simplified way with her growing interest in technology, specifically computers. She came across an article on the new role of the informatics nurse and began imagining herself doing that. Exactly what she would be doing and where was vague, but the more she imagined it and allowed for the possibility of it, the more motivated she felt about exploring what it would take to make it happen.

When she heard that the hospital was offering computer classes, she jumped at the chance to enroll. She also volunteered to work on a newly formed taskforce that was designing self-taught computer modules for patients. Her dissatisfaction with her current job was easier to tolerate because she used every opportunity to add to the skills and competencies she believed were transferable to her future vision. She volunteered to assist in the development of standardized teaching plans to make the work of busy nurses easier. She found resources for and developed patient teaching kits with handouts that simplified concepts and saved time. As she was doing this, she pored over the want ads to learn what the qualifications were for informatics nurses, what kind of organizations employed them, and what kind of educational preparation was required. She read everything she could get her hands on about this role, attended seminars about it, and eventually entered a graduate program that prepared nurses for it. Clarissa used her vision to encourage her to move forward as she strengthened her mission and held tight to her values. In this way she made productive and creative use of an otherwise unacceptable employment situation.

Creating a vision relies mostly on the thinking style most closely associated with the right brain, where thought occurs in mental impressions, fleeting images, and intuitive hunches. It is the twin partner to the logical processing and sequential reasoning associated with left brain thinking capacities. Using both of these capacities results in a more complete picture of your career future. While considering your future with left brain capacities leads to goals, tasks, and checklists, considering the future using your right brain can be a way to encourage and even accelerate momentum toward your dreams and hopes. This can often serve to encourage you so that the difficulties sometimes inherent in the fulfillment of your mission and values do not overwhelm or discourage you.

Right-brain thought is rich with the information and also the support needed to move into the future, but because rational reasoning is favored as the dominant thinking style of the scientifically based Western world, our right brain receives less training and validation. Creative right brain activities are not always understood or encouraged. As a child, you may remember daydreaming (an essential function of creativity and vision building) and being told by a parent or teacher that you were not paying attention. Or perhaps you were told not to let your imagination run away with you as you wrote a story or spoke to an imaginary playmate. These normal, creative, and eminently useful right-brain thinking processes can be recaptured by devoting a little time and effort to relearning and remembering them, and by suspending judgment and criticism of the process as well as the results.

Tips and Guidelines for Developing Your Vision

Write It Down

Write down your vision and recall it frequently. Then say it aloud, to yourself at first, always using present-tense vocabulary. Writing it down creates a kind of contract with yourself, and speaking about it in the present tense acts as a feedback loop to strengthen it and your resolve when the going gets tough. Share it with people who encourage and believe in you. Hearing yourself talk about it out loud reinforces the reality of it and helps move it from the possible to the probable, and eventually into the actual.

Take Your Vision Outside of Your Comfort Zone

Allow your vision to stretch you beyond your comfort zone without being unrealistic or overly ambitious. Marcia Perkins-Reed writes about vision in her book, *Thriving in Transition*. She says:

> "It should challenge us to reach further than we have before. If we do this at each of our transitional junctures, we will be constantly growing into greater possibilities. So if we think we can easily earn $45,000 in our next position, a minimum salary of $47,500 or $50,000 should appear in our vision statement. While we don't want to push ourselves relentlessly, ever striving towards elusive new goals that we don't believe will bring us success, we do want to expand our vision into the highest and best situation we can imagine knowing that what we attract may be even better than that!"[4]

Don't Let Stress Be an Obstacle

Tolerate the tension that naturally exists between your future vision and your present reality. Robert Fritz in *The Path of Least Resistance* describes this as essential to the creative process that will eventually manifest your vision. He suggests that it is necessary to hold in your mind the simultaneous experiences of how you want your life to be and how your life actually is now. The gap between these two experiences will narrow in favor of the path that offers the least resistance. Managing the stress created by the tension between your present reality and your future vision is necessary to support your movement forward, rather than allow your vision to collapse into your present reality.[5]

Be Patient

Don't expect your vision to occur immediately or to be crystal clear. Clarity will emerge over time as the experiences you have along the way shape and enhance the vision further. It may take a while to arrive at your vision, as you review and revise it over the time it takes to get there. In truth, for those who learn to use this kind of visionary skill, arrival is a short-lived experience on the way to a continually evolving future always just tantalizingly out of reach. Your vision, like your life, is an ever-unfolding process, a journey over time, not necessarily a destination. Learning to relish the experience of getting there as much as the arrival is an excellent way to approach life in constant transition and rapid change. This does not mean that goals are never achieved, but rather that where you have arrived is always a step to what is next.

Stay Focused on the Future

Reflect frequently on the question, "Where do you see yourself in the future? Doing what, with whom?" Consider starting a journal to capture and track the progressive development of your vision, using it as encouragement and motivation. Or carry a small notebook with you to capture fleeting thoughts or images related to your evolving vision. Often, when you turn your attention away from something you've been pondering, clarity emerges unexpectedly and spontaneously.

A Vision Exercise

Everyone has the capacity to visualize. The more you practice this ability, the stronger it will become. In some ways, visualizing is just another way of thinking, which you do more often than you realize. To demonstrate this, bring to mind your living room. Take about 15 seconds to recall the room and its contents, including any colors, associated sounds, or even aromas or physical sensations.

Most likely you thought about your living room not in words but in images, or more specifically in mental impressions of where the furniture and objects of your living room were. Perhaps you even had some associated sensory experiences like the sound of birds outside your window. In bringing to mind your living room, you most likely imagined it, visualized it, saw it on the movie screen of your mind. In the same way, you can create images of your future, and see yourself there. You can start by doing the exercise that follows. See Print Resources at the back of this book for additional resources.

A Vision of Your Future Self

Step 1:   Begin by sitting quietly in a comfortable place where you won't be interrupted for about 30 minutes.

Step 2:   Prepare yourself by performing a breathing or relaxation exercise that quiets your mind, allows you to turn inward, and creates a receptive attitude within you. (See Print Resources at the back of this book for suggested breathing and relaxation exercises.)

Step 3:   Reflect on the following questions and allow the answers to form as images or mental impressions on the movie screen of your mind rather than in words:

What are you doing? With whom?

In one year?

In five years?

In ten years?

In any future time?

What sounds, sensations, feelings arise?

Keep the emphasis on imagining your self and what is going on around you and within you. Avoid developing a mental list of plans and tasks so that you can stimulate the right brain creative process rather than left brain problem-solving.

Step 4:   Answer the following questions and then use these answers to form your vision statement. Reflect on this frequently, pondering it over time, and allowing it to shape and reshape itself.

How I see myself in the future:_____

What I am doing: _____

Who I am with:_____

Where I am and what is around me: _____

What I hear and feel around me and within me: _____

WHAT DO YOU HAVE TO OFFER?

Now that you know a bit more about who you are, let's turn our attention to the second of the two components that determine your product/service, namely, what you have to offer. To know this, you need to be clear about what you are good at and what you prefer to spend most of your working time doing. Because there are so many nursing roles and practice possibilities, you may find it difficult to determine what is best for you. An approach that can provide clarity is to understand how nursing roles contain specific work skills and activities that are blended with the core competencies that every nurse has. Even though nursing roles resist strict categorization, this approach provides a good enough general direction, which you can personalize and strengthen by combining the role with your mission, your vision, and your values/needs.

Nursing roles are extremely fluid; they are often influenced by the unique patient care needs in a particular setting. While each nurse is accountable to the standard of practice described in the Nurse Practice Act, to some degree the functions of the role are open to the interpretation of the nurse performing it. Nursing roles are also responsive to organizational policies as well as to marketplace trends and changes. Hence, a nurse manager in one setting might work very differently from a nurse manager in another setting. Likewise, the job description for a medical-surgical staff nurse will look different in a community hospital than it does in a major medical center.

Blending Basic Work Activities with Core Competencies in Nursing

Combining your preference for specific work activities with the core competencies necessary to perform them creates a nursing role. Since basic work activities and core competencies are rarely performed in isolation from one another, the overlap that exists when describing them is reflective of the creative complexity inherent in nursing practice.

YOUR NURSING ROLE IS A BLENDING OF:		
Basic work skills +	Core nursing competencies =	Your nursing role
May include several categories of skills, with one or more in dominant use	May include more than one competency, with one or more being used primarily	Direct care nurse, or nurse manager, or staff development specialist, etc.

There are three generally recognized categories of work activities performed by the nurse. These are best described as skills and activities involving (1) *people*, (2) *data and information*, and (3) *concepts and ideas*. The box on the next page specifies what may comprise each of these three major categories of work skills.

The five generally recognized core competencies inherent in the nursing role are: (1) *clinical expertise*, (2) *managerial expertise*, (3) *educational expertise*, (4) *interpersonal expertise*, and (5) *technical expertise*. Each of these is described in greater detail in the following pages.

BASIC WORK SKILLS

People Skills	Data and Information Skills	Concept and Idea Skills
counseling	systematizing	creating
motivating	using logic	translating
advocating	classifying information	visualizing
empathizing	analyzing facts	conceptualizing
coaching	compiling information	synthesizing
persuading	summarizing	inventing
facilitating	working with numbers	designing
delegating	testing hypothesis	symbolizing
training	allocating resources	acting
teaching	keeping records	innovating
listening	tabulating	extrapolating
advising	budgeting	demonstrating
interviewing	keeping inventories	communicating
resolving conflicts	using logic	evaluating
collaborating	editing	presenting
providing	mediating	reviewing
performing	negotiating	assisting
assessing	informing	developing
appreciating	regulating	interpreting
intervening	assigning	imagining
accomplishing	appreciating	affecting
alleviating	combining	affirming
defending	directing	confirming
enhancing	devising	empowering
healing	gathering	encouraging
improving	generating	fostering
nurturing	manifesting	illuminating
safeguarding	revising	involving
supporting	planning	persuading
sustaining	progressing	praising
touching	validating	translating

Clinical Competencies

These competencies describe the direct relationship a nurse has with a patient. It involves using specific technical skills within the nursing process of (1) assessing patient needs and responses, (2) planning the patient's care, (3) intervening with actions as required and necessary, and (4) evaluating the outcome of actions taken. The goal of the nurse employing these clinical competencies is to influence, support, or sustain a patient's physical, emotional, mental, spiritual, or interpersonal needs. All nurses who provide direct patient care utilize clinical competencies as well as the other four nursing competencies (described below). Likewise, many of the work activities related to people, data, and information, as well as concepts and ideas are frequently represented in these clinical nursing competencies and are expressed in a variety of clinical nursing roles. Examples of clinical competencies typically performed in the clinical role of the medical surgical nurse at the novice or expert level might be:

- Caring for postoperative patients
- Inserting IV lines
- Counseling families of dying patients
- Calculating medications
- Planning for discharge
- Teaching self-care to patients
- Interpreting data from monitor readouts
- Mentoring new nurses

Interpersonal Competencies

These competencies involve communicating with and relating to others. They often reflect—but are not limited to—the basic activities involved in people skills and concept and idea skills. Since clinical competencies cannot exist without interpersonal competencies, some of the examples from above could just as easily be used here, such as teaching self-care to patients, mentoring new nurses, and counseling families of dying patients. Additional examples might include:

- Conducting medication teaching groups
- Empathizing with an anxious patient
- Collaborating with physicians
- Actively listening to a family member's concern

- Advocating for patients' rights
- Resolving conflicts between home health aides

Managerial Competencies

These competencies primarily involve planning, organizing, directing, and controlling system resources as well as the people in them. Data and information skills are often correlated with managerial competencies. General managerial competencies are part of the role of the nurse providing direct patient care, as well as the nurse manager who oversees it. Examples include:

- Supervising nursing staff
- Conducting studies of sick time utilization
- Writing annual performance evaluations
- Writing handbooks for patient care technicians
- Using computers to develop budgets
- Designing new patient care delivery system
- Coordinating patient care activities
- Delegating responsibilities to others

Educational Competencies

These competencies primarily involve communicating concepts and ideas to others by means of explaining, teaching, and coaching. Once again, educational competencies are closely related to all the other nursing competencies, including, of course, interpersonal competencies. Examples include:

- Teaching CPR to new mothers
- Teaching glucometer use to diabetic patients
- Designing nursing school curricula
- Creating orientation programs
- Mentoring new graduates
- Presenting online learning programs

Technical Competencies

These competencies involve the use of equipment and machinery, often complex and computerized, in correlation with other nursing competencies. Technical competencies rely heavily on the basic work abilities of data and information skills, and cut across all nursing roles, in one way or another. High-tech and low-tech examples include:

- Regulating ventilators
- Presenting online learning programs
- Taking blood pressures
- Hemodynamic monitoring
- Obtaining blood samples from central IV lines
- Using computers to input lab data
- Performing wound care
- Using computers to develop budgets

The Colors of Your Nursing Palette

Just as the primary colors of red, yellow, and blue form the basis of a vast color palate, so does the blending of these basic work skills with the core nursing competencies determine the "color" of your nursing practice palate. Nurses who prefer people skills make excellent direct care nurses at the novice or expert level as they develop the work skills that accompany this role. This role may vary among different workplaces and might include a higher or lower proportion of data and information skills or concept and idea skills. Likewise nurses with a high preference for data and information skills make good managers, and generally speaking, nurses with a high preference for concept and idea skills could make good nurse educators.

By blending these work skills and nursing competencies you can create a career pathway to one or more of the clinical, administrative, educational, research, and consulting options in nursing practice and/or in the healthcare industry in general. See the box on the next page for more examples of nursing roles, and see the back of this book for additional resources on nursing roles and career profiles. Chapter 11, "The Market Research Department of *You, Inc.*" will elaborate on these roles and discuss the healthcare environments in which they can be found.

**EXAMPLES OF NURSING ROLES CORRELATED WITH
CORE COMPETENCIES AND BASIC WORK SKILLS**

Clinical Competencies

Direct care nurse

Adult nurse practitioner

Psychiatric clinical nurse specialist

Community health nurse

Telephone triage nurse

Managerial Competencies

Nurse manager in a cardiac care center

Vice president, nursing and patient care
   services

Nurse researcher

Case manager

Educational Competencies

Staff development specialist

Professor, college of nursing

Community health educator

Childbirth educator

Interpersonal Competencies

Parish nurse

Bereavement counselor

Addictions and substance abuse
specialist

Nurse psychotherapist

Technical Competencies

Informatics nurse

Critical care nurse

High tech home care nurse

Sales representative for high tech company

Levels of Nursing Proficiency

Another factor to consider in determining what you have to offer is your current level of proficiency. Pat Benner's classic and oft-quoted work, *From Novice to Expert,* is useful in making this self-assessment, and then ultimately helpful in determining whether this level of proficiency meets the requirements of your current or future employer. As discussed in Chapter 5, "The Newly Graduated Nurse," Benner describes the five stages each nursing role has at the novice, advanced beginner, competent, proficient, and expert levels.[6]

A novice has no experience in the role to be performed; for example, the newly graduated nurse or nurse practitioner. The advanced beginner has limited, recurring experience; for example, a new B.S.N. graduate with nine months experience on a medical-surgical unit. The level called competent describes a nurse who has at least two years of experience performing the same role. At the level Brenner calls proficient, the nurse can practice in situations requiring greater speed and flexibility, generally thought to occur after performing the role for three to five years. Nurses practicing at the expert level have achieved an intuitive and immediate level of mastery in complex situations thought to occur after a period of five or more years of experience in the same role.

Each time you move between the generic roles of clinician, manager, or educator, there may be a need to move through these proficiency levels again. You will bring to your new role what you've learned along the way in the form of transferable skills, abilities, and experiences. While this may help you move up the hierarchy in your new role, the very act of practicing in a new role can lead to some insecurity. You might feel uncomfortable unless you come to understand the need to progress along this learning curve through to the next proficiency level.

Take Karen, for example. An ANCC board-certified (at the generalist level) medical-surgical staff nurse with ten years of experience in a variety of inpatient and ambulatory settings, including critical care, Karen is practicing at the expert level according to Benner's model. Upon graduation from the adult nurse practitioner program that she has been attending for the last two years, she could be considered a novice in that role and will need to give herself time to progress again through the levels of nursing practice proficiency. A lack of tolerance for this necessary transition can result in a loss of confidence that might prevent Karen from seeking employment as a nurse practitioner.

Professional Certification

To be board certified at either the general practice level or at the specialist level announces and advertises to the healthcare marketplace your pride in meeting the high standards established by the nursing profession. Every business owner, including, of course, *You, Inc.,* would want to utilize this kind of product development and recognition to his or her benefit.

The American Nurses Credentialing Center (ANCC) is an arm of the American Nurses Association and offers board certification at the generalist and specialist levels in the following areas of nursing practice:

- Medicine and surgery
- Gerontology
- Pediatrics
- Perinatal, Ob-Gyn
- Community health
- Psychiatric/Mental health

ANCC also offers the very prestigious Magnet status certification to healthcare organizations that have met certain standards of excellence. These Magnet status organizations have standards and criteria that insure quality patient care as well as nursing practice environments that foster professional satisfaction. Some of the ways in which *You, Inc.* can take advantage of this Magnet status include:

- Seek employment in Magnet status organizations.
- Identify your association with a Magnet status facility on your resume.
- Find an appropriate way to mention this association in an interview.
- Determine if your present organization plans to apply for Magnet status. Consider suggesting this, including how it would benefit patient care.
- Work on committees in your organization if it is seeking Magnet status. (Be sure to include this on your resume.)
- Network with nurses who work in Magnet status organizations, especially when you are considering seeking employment there.

Certification in many nursing specialties is also available. Some of the professional associations that offer certification include:

Nursing Specialty	Professional Association
Critical Care Nursing (CCRN)	American Association of Critical Care Nurses
Occupational Health Nursing (COHN)	American Board for Occupational Health Nurses
Emergency Nursing (CEN)	Board of Certification for Emergency Nursing
Infection Control Nursing (CIC)	Certification Board of Infection Control

See Internet Resources at the back of this book for additional certification resources.

CHAPTER **11**

The Market Research
Department of *You, Inc.*

Of the many influences on the healthcare marketplace in these early years of the new millennium, two are most profound: the crisis of the nursing shortage and the continuing healthcare revolution begun in the 1990s resulting in the restructuring of the healthcare system.

That a shortage of nurses exists translates into amazing opportunities for every nurse working today and everyone who wants to become a nurse. All crises are turning points ripe with possibilities for something different, something new and better. Healthcare is a growth industry and since nurses work everywhere in healthcare, the marketplace is a rich landscape for the Nurse CEO of *You, Inc.*

The managed care era that began in the 1990s brought economic restraint and cost containment, and created a revolution in healthcare delivery services whose repercussions are still reverberating in this new millennium—and the dust hasn't settled yet. The enormous challenges yet to be addressed in meeting the healthcare needs of American citizens—aging baby boomers; access to healthcare, insurance and prescription coverage; the rising cost of healthcare services; protection against bioterrorism—will shake the foundation of the healthcare industry in ways yet to be seen, surely affecting where and how nurses work.

THE 21st-CENTURY HEALTHCARE ENVIRONMENT

The "hospitalcentric" age of healthcare based on the medical model, which focused on taking care of patients who were ill or injured, is ending. In its place is evolving a "continuum of care," a framework for the delivery of healthcare services that focuses on health maintenance as well as illness and injury. While hospitals took care of patients from admission to discharge, the continuum of care addresses the healthcare needs of people (who may sometimes become patients) from birth to death.

The continuum of care represents a paradigm shift, a sea change in healthcare delivery, with a movement from problem-oriented medical diagnosis and cure to a perspective on holism, prevention, and self-care. In this continuum, patients receive care along a pathway that spans the gamut between wellness and prevention of illness on one end, to rehabilitation, long-term care, and end-of-life care on the other end, all of which greatly broadens employment opportunities for nurses. Characteristics of this newly emerging healthcare system include the following, as enumerated by Vivien DeBack in "The New Practice Environment" in *Nurse Case Management in the 21st Century.*

- An emphasis on health, prevention, and wellness, with an attention to risk factors, along with the expectation that people will take more responsibility for their health.
- Intensive use of and reliance on information systems for patient documentation and for access to current practice information.
- Reconsideration of human values, with careful assessment of the balance between the expanding capability of technology and the need for humane treatment.
- Focus on consumer and patient satisfaction, with the encouragement of patient partnerships in decisions related to treatment.
- Knowledge of treatment outcomes with emphasis on the most effective treatment under different conditions.
- Constrained resources, with cost containment to limit expenditures.
- Coordination of resources, with an emphasis on teams to improve efficiency.
- Growing awareness of the domestic and global healthcare issues of health, education, and public safety.[1]

EMPLOYMENT TRENDS AND PREDICTIONS

Even though the hospital will remain the largest employment setting for nurses, the kind of work nurses do in hospitals will center around caring for the sickest patients, frequently for the shortest length of stay, with recovery continuing for these patients elsewhere along the continuum of care. This will create a dramatic increase in employment opportunities, especially as the healthcare needs of the American people continue to increase as predicted.

The U.S. Department of Labor *(Occupational Outlook Handbook, 2002–3 Edition, dol. gov)* identifies the following significant factors related to the healthcare marketplace, expected to affect the employment of registered nurses:

Employment Trends

- Registered nurses represent the largest healthcare occupation, with more than two million jobs.
- The profession of nursing is one of the ten occupations projected to have the largest numbers of new jobs; job opportunities are expected to be very good.
- Earnings are above average, particularly for advanced practice nurses who have additional education or training.
- About three out of five jobs are in hospital inpatient and outpatient departments.
- Hospital nurses form the largest group of nurses.
- Other nurses (one out of four were part time) are employed in:
    —offices and clinics of physicians and other healthcare practitioners
    —home healthcare agencies
    —nursing homes
    —temporary help agencies
    —schools
    —government agencies
    —residential care facilities
    —social service agencies
    —religious organizations

—research facilities

—management and public relations firms

—insurance agencies

—private households

Job Outlook

- The job outlook for registered nurses is classified as "very good," meaning that job openings as compared to job seekers may be more numerous.

- Employment of nurses is expected to "grow faster than the average," with employment projected to increase 21–35 percent for all occupations through 2010.

- Because the occupation is very large, many new jobs will result.

- Thousands of job openings will result from the need to replace experienced nurses who will be leaving the occupation, especially as the median age of the registered nurse population continues to rise.

- Some states report current and projected shortages of R.N.s, primarily due to an aging workforce and recent declines in nursing school enrollments. Imbalances between supply of and demand for qualified workers should spur efforts to attract and retain qualified R.N.s. For example, employers may restructure workloads, improve compensation and working conditions, and/or subsidize training or continuing education.

- Faster than average growth will be driven by technological advances in patient care, which permit a greater number of medical problems to be treated, and an increasing emphasis on preventative care. In addition, the number of older people, who are much more likely than younger people to need nursing care, is projected to grow rapidly.

- Employment in hospitals, the largest sector, is expected to grow more slowly than in other healthcare sectors. While the intensity of nursing care is likely to increase, requiring more nurses per patient, the number of inpatients (those who remain in the hospital for more than 24 hours) is not likely to increase much. Patients are being discharged earlier and more procedures are being done on an outpatient basis, both in and outside hospitals.

- Rapid growth is expected in hospital outpatient facilities, such as those providing same-day surgery, rehabilitation, and chemotherapy.

- Employment in home healthcare is expected to grow rapidly. This is in response to the growing number of older persons with functional disabilities, consumer preference for care in the home, and the technological advances that make it possible to bring increasingly complex treatments into the home. The type of care demanded would require nurses who are able to perform complex procedures.

- Employment in nursing homes is expected to grow faster than average due to an increase in the number of elderly, many of whom require long-term care. In addition, the financial pressure on hospitals to discharge patients as soon as possible should produce more nursing home admissions.

- Growth in agencies that provide specialized long-term rehabilitation for stroke and head injury patients or that treat Alzheimer's victims will increase employment.

- An increasing proportion of sophisticated procedures, which once were performed only in hospitals, are being performed in physician's offices and clinics, including ambulatory surgicenters and emergency medical centers. Accordingly, employment is expected to grow faster than average in these places as healthcare in general expands.

- In evolving integrated healthcare networks, nurses may rotate among employment settings. Because jobs in traditional hospital nursing positions are no longer the only option, R.N.s will need to be flexible. Opportunities should be excellent, particularly for nurses with advanced education and training.

- Individuals considering nursing (and those nurses with diplomas or associate degrees) should consider enrolling in a B.S.N. program because, if they do so, their advancement opportunities usually are broader. In fact, some career paths are open only to nurses with bachelor's or advanced degrees. A bachelor's degree is often necessary for administrative positions, and it is a prerequisite for admission to graduate nursing programs in research, consulting, teaching, or a clinical specialization.[2]

MAKING THE BEST USE OF TRENDS AND PREDICTIONS

Are you excited yet? What a fantastic time to be a nurse! No matter what generation of nursing you belong to, whether novice or expert, whatever your specialty or your preference for healthcare setting, there is a place for you in the current and emerging healthcare marketplace. Not ready to retire yet? Don't! Nursing needs you! Want to work in critical care but you just graduated? No problem! Seek out the extended orientation and training programs offered by many employers who need to train their own critical care nurses because they can't find enough of them to fill all the vacancies they have.

Nurses who want to make the best use of these exciting trends and predictions will keep the following in mind:

- Unless you are interested in the fast-paced, high-tech environment of acute care hospitals where relationships with patients is short-term, seek employment elsewhere among the vast opportunities along the continuum of care.
- Nurses with a B.S.N. and advanced education will be seen as best qualified by most employers.
- Watch for and take advantage of training and education subsidized by employers and government agencies.
- Seek out employers who are aware of the need to restructure roles and staffing patterns, as well as the need to improve working conditions to attract and retain nurses.
- Stay ahead of your technological learning curve. No nurse anywhere along the continuum of care can get by without some level of comfort around healthcare technology as well as at least a beginning level of computer literacy. *While you may be able to choose low-tech vs high-tech care, there is no longer any such thing as "no-tech."*
- Consider aligning your career path with emerging healthcare needs, trends, and predictions, for example, informatics, eldercare, or homeland security focused on preparing first responders to terrorism attacks.
- Take your self-care seriously to ensure that you have the resilience and stamina needed to manage the rigors and demands of this exciting profession, and to prevent burnout.

BECOMING A TREND-WATCHER

Stay tuned; keep current; watch the trends. Don't allow *You, Inc.* to be without the information it needs to take advantage of what's new and what's next! Take the warning of futurists and forecasters seriously when they say that a *change affecting the way you live and work will occur every six months.*

To obtain the most up-to-date information about the healthcare marketplace, access the websites and home pages of professional associations and organizations, as well as government bureaus and agencies. Develop the habit of checking in frequently with your favorite online nursing networking site (you do have one, don't you?). To the recommendations that follow, add your own and see the Resources at the back of this book for additional sites and resources.

Professional and Government Organizations

- U.S. Department of Labor: *www.dol.gov*
- Bureau of Labor Statistics: *www.bls.gov*
- National League for Nurses: *www.nln.org*
- American Association for Colleges in Nursing: *www.aacn.nche.edu*
- American Nurses Association: *www.nursingworld.org*

Online Nursing Networks and Career Information Sites

- *HospitalSoup.com*
- *CyberNurse.com*
- *Nursing.advanceweb.com/main.aspx*
- *UltimateNurse.com*
- *NursingSpectrum.com*

Your own list of trend-watching and networking websites:

_____   _____

_____   _____

_____   _____

NURSING PRACTICE SETTINGS ALONG THE CONTINUUM OF CARE

Along the continuum of care are the healthcare options for patients, along with employment opportunities for the nurse of today and tomorrow. An overview of the continuum of care includes the following nursing practice environments:

Acute-Care Hospitals

This is among the most familiar of the facilities along the continuum of care, where most people believe they will go when ill or injured and where the majority of nurses will continue to work, but as described above, differently than in generations past. Nurses in this extremely fluid, high-tech environment will see fast-paced action, rapid turnover of acutely or critically ill patients, and short-term relationships with patients.

Post-Acute-Care Facilities and Services

Post-acute-care services are among the fastest growing sectors along the continuum of care and include transitional hospitals, subacute-care facilities, long-term care facilities (previously called nursing homes), assisted living facilities, home healthcare services, and adult day-care agencies.

Transitional Hospitals

These facilities, which are relatively new on the continuum of care, provide longer-term care for acutely ill patients who are in stable condition. The patients in these facilities require intensive, skilled care from a wide variety of healthcare disciplines, with the average minimum stay around 25 days. Following his horseback riding accident, the actor Christopher Reeve was cared for in a transitional hospital after he was stabilized in an acute-care hospital.

Because the transitional hospital doesn't have to fund services typically found in acute-care hospitals such as ambulatory clinics and emergency departments, they can provide a broad range of acute-care interventions, including ICU-type services at about one-third to one-half the cost of acute care hospitals. This, of course, makes them quite attractive to managed-care companies. Rather than duplicate such services as lab and x-ray, they purchase them when needed from affiliated agencies, thereby avoiding the costly purchase and maintenance of these services. This is a great practice environment for the nurse who enjoys high-tech, acute/critical care but wants a longer-term relationship with patients, and enjoys a strong emphasis on teaching and patient self-care.

Subacute-Care Facilities

The patient requiring care in subacute facilities falls somewhere between needing less intensive care than an acute-care hospital would provide but more than what the long-term facility can offer. This, along with rehabilitation, makes for a unique combination of services. The care provided is short-term (average length of stay is five to fourteen days), with a focused plan geared to helping the patient achieve a specific goal, for example, walk independently with a cane following hip replacement surgery. The patient is referred to the next place along the continuum of care, as indicated. These patients are stable, but can still be quite ill, often requiring high-tech monitoring. As in the transitional hospital, they receive skilled interventions from a multidisciplinary team.

Long-Term Care Facilities

The change in name from nursing home to long-term care facility reflects the influence of changing economics and reimbursement mechanisms. These facilities restructured their services in response to the need to provide a higher level of skilled intervention for their patients when they became ill, rather than transferring them to more costly facilities like acute care hospitals. In addition to being an extension of the patient's family and community that it has always been, the long-term care facility now has an increasing number of specialty units, all designed to treat the patient while ill. Examples include dementia and AIDS care.

Hospice Services

The majority of hospice services are part of and administered by home care programs, or by inpatient facilities along the continuum of care, such as the acute-care hospital, in collaboration with the home-care agency's visiting nurses. Hospice care provides services and support to terminally ill patients (generally with a prognosis of six months or less to live), including skilled nursing care, home health aides and attendants, and specialized medical equipment as indicated. The combined focus on physical care and emotional support is frequently described by hospice nurses as both rewarding and challenging.

Assisted Living Facilities

This relatively new and mostly privately funded addition to the continuum of care provides several levels of healthcare and personal care services for the well elderly who want to live independently, as well as special facilities for the frail elderly. Other groups, such as the physically and emotionally disabled, are starting to take advantage of this new option. Assisted living facilities offer apartment-style living along with such personal support as dining room meals, often served in attractive restaurant-like atmospheres, household cleaning and repair, and recreational activities. The residents enjoy the benefits of security, companionship, and access to ongoing healthcare, or if necessary, emergency care. Ambulatory or inpatient care, when needed, is provided through a network of affiliated agencies, often representing all the options along the care continuum. Even patients with dementia and Alzheimer's disease can be accommodated in the specialized units of some assisted living facilities.

Home Healthcare Services

Technological advances as well as economic restraints have fostered a boom in home healthcare services. This is believed to be the fastest growing segment of the healthcare marketplace, with high-tech home care and psychiatric home care growing the fastest. Today's homecare patient tends to be more severely or chronically ill than ever before. Home care agencies fall into three general categories: licensed, certified, and long-term:

- The licensed agencies provide private-duty nursing as well as assistive and personal care support, often from home health attendants.
- The certified agencies care for sicker patients, often those discharged "sicker and quicker" from acute care hospitals, and offer a broad range of services such as rehabilitation, assistance in daily living activities from home health aides, and social service support.
- Long-term home care agencies provide supportive care to those patients who are chronically ill and qualify for a long-term, inpatient care facility but who chose to remain at home.

Adult Day-Care Services

These facilities provide skilled nursing, assisted personal care, and long-term care to patients that may or may not be receiving simultaneous home care services. Patients come to day-care for socialization or for such skilled nursing services as insulin monitoring and tracheostomy care. These facilities provide the patients with an enhanced quality of life, and the caregiver-relative with an excellent option for rest and relief, or just the freedom to do errands or go to work.

Community-Based Services

These familiar healthcare facilities have long existed in the community, outside the traditional walls of acute-care hospitals. Community-based healthcare services are increasing in number, with a growing variety of responses to the new model of healthcare within the continuum of care. These services include:

- Ambulatory healthcare centers, including physician or nurse-based practices, free-standing or hospital-based clinics, and health maintenance organizations for all healthcare specialties, including mental health and substance abuse
- Ambulatory surgicenters
- Occupational and corporate healthcare services and wellness programs found in most traditional workplaces as well as more exotic locations like movie sets, circuses, sporting events, concerts, resorts, camps, spas, health clubs, and weight loss centers
- Family planning centers
- Birthing centers
- Pain management centers
- Wound care centers
- Hemodialysis centers
- Outreach centers of churches, synagogues, and other religious institutions
- Forensic and prison healthcare services and facilities
- School health offices and centers
- Shelters, housing assistance, and mobile crisis programs for the homeless and mentally ill

Supporting and/or Affiliating Services

Completing most of the picture of nursing practice options that relate directly or indirectly to the continuum of care are the facilities, services, institutions, and organizations described below. These form a web of support that serves and/or affiliates with the care continuum, including institutions for the education of healthcare personnel. These services may represent the for-profit and nonprofit sectors and include:

- **Pharmaceutical and medical supply companies**. These companies hire nurses to market their products to a variety of healthcare organizations and agencies. Competencies required might include teaching skills and knowledge of the product, for example, the use of specialized dressings for wound care.
- **Healthcare consulting organizations**. These include a vast array of services and programs including computer consulting, organizational redesign experts, healthcare accrediting organizations, and so on.
- **Personnel supply agencies** that provide professional and ancillary staff to healthcare organizations.
- **Schools and colleges** for the education of nurses and other healthcare personnel.

21st-CENTURY NURSING COMPETENCIES

Nurse CEOs of *You, Inc.* recognize the need to develop the following nursing competencies, knowing that there is an increased emphasis on them in the models of healthcare emerging in the 21st century:

- Advocacy for patients or anyone accessing healthcare services
- Teaching, learning, and coaching
- Collaboration and increased teamwork
- Resource management
- Critical thinking
- Flexibility in thinking and acting
- Relational and communication skills for collaborative team practice
- Information management skills
- Keen sensitivity to and support of cultural diversity
- Community health and systems perspectives

NURSING ROLES AND EMPLOYMENT ALONG THE CONTINUUM OF CARE

Now that you are armed with a map of healthcare's territories, you can consider the nursing roles and employment options associated with them. As healthcare continues to evolve and restructure its services along the continuum of care, nursing roles and responsibilities will evolve as well.

The three generic roles of direct care nurse, nurse-manager, and nurse-educator, at the basic or advanced levels of practice, and at the novice as well as the expert levels of proficiency, can be found in a variety of employment venues, with the potential for many future options and opportunities.

On the next pages, these generic nursing roles are combined with examples of nursing practice options and potential places of employment along the continuum of care. This is certainly not an all-inclusive list but does represent a way to think about the vast employment opportunities available to you.

The best way for you to explore these options and determine your interest in and qualifications for them is to access online information about them. A second option is to talk to other nurses who are working in these roles, through online or in-person networking. Nursing websites that you might find helpful are listed earlier in this chapter under the headings "Professional and Government Organizations" and "Online Nursing Networks and Career Information Sites," as well as in Chapter 4, "The Nurse and Technology." The Resources at the back of this book contain additional sites and print resources as well. Asterisks indicate nursing practice options related to recent trends and needs.

GENERIC NURSING ROLE	EXAMPLE OF NURSING PRACTICE OPTION	POTENTIAL PLACE OF EMPLOYMENT ALONG THE CONTINUUM OF CARE
Manager Educator	Informatics nurse*	All settings
Educator	Nursing school faculty	Colleges and schools of nursing Continuing education sites
Manager	Nurse case manager	Inpatient settings
Direct care nurse	Risk alert manager	Community settings
	Utilization review nurse	Insurance companies
Direct care nurse	Medical-surgical nurse	Acute-care hospital
Direct care nurse	Telephone triage nurse*	Managed care companies Insurance companies Hospital EDs
Direct care nurse	Parish nurse	Churches, religious centers
Direct care nurse Manager Educator	Infection control nurse*	Private and government agencies of homeland security for protection against bioterrorism attacks

GENERIC NURSING ROLE	EXAMPLE OF NURSING PRACTICE OPTION	POTENTIAL PLACE OF EMPLOYMENT ALONG THE CONTINUUM OF CARE
Direct care nurse	Nurse consultant	Pharmaceutical companies
		Hospital supply companies
		Private practice
Direct care nurse	Nurse attorney	Private practice
Manager	Legal nurse consultant	Attorney's office
Educator	Paralegal nurse	Risk management departments in all settings
Direct care nurse Manager	Nurse entrepreneur	Private practice in psychotherapy
Educator		Owner of home care agency
Direct care nurse	Advanced practice nurse	Nurse-run clinic
	Nurse practitioner	Nurse-physician group practice
	Clinical nurse specialist	All settings as primary care provider

To obtain more information about where and how nurses work, consider online resources, such as The Student Nurse Forum (*kcsun3.tripod.com*). It provides support, information, resources, and advice to nursing students about education and practice, and has a very fine section on career profiles for many nursing roles ("60 specialty areas and counting!"), including those lesser known. What makes this presentation of nursing roles stand out from many others is its accompanying links to articles on the Internet "that are first-person in nature and give you a feel for what a 'day in the life' would be." A sampling of what they provide follows. Roles that are new and/or represent the changing focus in healthcare are marked with an asterisk:

NURSING ROLE	CAREER PROFILE	WEBSITE
Medical-Surgical Nurse	"A Walk on the Wild Side"	*nurseweek.com*
Burn Unit Nurse	"Burn Nurses Travel to New York to Help Victims"	*www.mc.vanderbilt.edu/reporter/?ID=1730*
Critical Care Nurse	"Critical Care Nurses"	*nursingworld.org*
Holistic Nurse*	"A New Attitude"	*nurseweek.com*
Home Health Nurse*	"Call Me If You Need Me"	*nursingspectrum.com*
Nurse Educator	"A Day in the Life: Nurse Educator"	*HospitalSoup.com*
Nurse Practitioner*	"P.N.P.'s Take Family Focus"	*nursingspectrum.com*
Informatics Nurse*	"A Day in the Life with Informatics Nurse Florence Valley"	*HospitalSoup.com*
Subacute Care Nurse*	"Subacute Care: A Growing Field of Practice For R.N.'s"	*nursingspectrum.com*
Telemedicine Nurse*	"Growing Pains"	*nurseweek.com*

There is every reason to be excited about the options and opportunities available for 21st-century nurses even though the challenges of nursing practice sometime make this difficult to hold on to. The following tips and strategies will help you achieve success in this exciting healthcare marketplace. Space is provided for you to list your own ideas for ensuring success:

- Work towards preserving a first class ticket to ride, a front row seat in the theatre of healthcare employment. This includes:
    - —A Bachelor of Science in nursing
    - —Professional certification at the generalist or specialist level
    - —Current and relevant continuing education
    - —Broad cross-training
    - —Superb self-care
- Stay loose and be flexible. Be prepared to move to what's new and what's next; revel in the adventure of it.
- See the opportunities and challenges rather than danger or threats in new work opportunities that come your way, whether expected or unexpected; manage the stress of change that often accompanies something new.
- Take your role as Nurse CEO of *You, Inc.* seriously. Develop a self-employed attitude, managing your career as if it was your own business, attending to all the departments of *You, Inc.* in ways that keep it aligned with the best employment options possible.
- Revise, revise, and revise again. Keep the root of the word *re-vise* in mind, which means "to see and to see again; to look over something; to correct or improve; to make a new version of; to take another look; to update." In relation to *You, Inc.*, this might mean to consider your mission, your vision, your resume, your nursing skills and competencies all works in progress, changing and evolving according to your professional and personal development in order to stay aligned with the current and emerging healthcare marketplace

Your strategies to ensure career success:

_____

_____

_____

CHAPTER 12

The Planning Department of *You, Inc.*

Like all successful business owners, the Nurse CEO of *You, Inc.* knows that a well-developed marketing plan is essential to success. Your marketing plan puts a foundation under your vision and translates your mission as a nurse into reality. The goals and their accompanying tasks become the pathway upon which you travel towards achieving what you once might have only dreamed or imagined. A well-thought out marketing plan reflects the special attributes of the work you do and helps you identify where it is most needed, where you would find the best match between your nursing skills and competencies and the healthcare marketplace. It takes the ideas and data generated from the other departments of *You, Inc.* and pulls them together into a coherent whole. Planning creates clarity and focus, essential for guiding yourself through the maze of employment options and the new workplace constant of rapid change.

A good marketing plan is a roadmap, a time schedule, and a feedback mechanism all rolled into one. When you add to this a measure of commitment and the encouragement and mentoring of people in your support network, you have a recipe for career success and resilience.

To develop your marketing plan, follow the steps in this chapter. Reflect on each section as it relates to your current or anticipated experience. Revisit and revise your plan periodically. You can expect to validate the marketability of your plan about every six months, since futurists and forecasters predict that changes affecting your work or personal life will most likely occur with that frequency.

STEP 1: DESCRIBE YOUR MISSION, YOUR VALUES, AND YOUR VISION

Your mission, values, and vision describe who you are as a nurse, and what you have to offer an employer. Together they represent what will give you career satisfaction and sustain you through the winds of change by grounding you in what is most meaningful and important to you, personally and professionally. Refer to your reflections in Chapter 10, "The Product Development Department of *You, Inc.*," and complete the following:

My Vision of Myself in Nursing

_____

My Mission in Nursing

Fill in the blanks below and then write your mission statement under it:

My mission (what I do):

_____, _____, and _____.

(your three verbs from Chapter 10, Step 1)

My values or principles (what I stand for):

_____

(your core values or principles from Step 2)

To or for, among or with (whom you help):

_____

(the group or cause from Step 3)

My mission statement is:

_____

_____

_____

My professional and personal values are:

_____

_____

_____

STEP 2: SELECT YOUR NURSING ROLE, YOUR "BUSINESS"

As discussed in Chapter 9, you own a business called *You, Inc.* This is your self-owned nursing practice of which you are the Nurse CEO. Your nursing practice "business" provides a service expressed in the nursing role you perform. Your nursing role is a blending of basic work skills and core nursing competencies. Refer to what you learned about your nursing role in Chapter 10 and then work through the steps that follow to identify the nursing role you currently have to offer a potential employer:

Basic Work Skills

1. Reflect on your present job, or one you may be considering.
2. List all the work skills and activities that this job requires.

_____

_____

3. Which skills and activities do you:

    like to do? _____

    dislike doing?_____

    want to do more of?_____

4. Refer to the general categories of basic work skills below. Which do you prefer to spend the most time doing? Rank them in your order of preference with 1 signifying "most preferred" and 3 signifying "least preferred":

    _____ People skills

    _____ Data and information skills

    _____ Concept and idea skills

Core Nursing Competencies

1. Refer to the discussion of core nursing competencies in Chapter 10, "The Product Development Department of *You, Inc.*" and the list below.

2. Which do you prefer to spend the most time doing? Rank them in your order of preference with 1 signifying most preferred and 3 signifying least preferred:

    _____ Clinical competencies

    _____ Managerial competencies

    _____ Educational competencies

    _____ Interpersonal competencies

    _____ Technical competencies

Your Preferred Nursing Role

The business you are currently in is: _____

An example of this role is: _____

Where a nurse in this example might work is (see Chapter 11, "The Market Research

Department of *You, Inc.*"): _____

STEP 3: ASSESS YOUR LEVEL OF NURSING PRACTICE PROFICIENCY

Using Benner's model as described in the Chapter 10, "The Product Development Department of *You, Inc.*," identify the level of nursing practice proficiency you have now, or the level that's expected in the role you are considering.[1]

- ❐ Level I = Novice
- ❐ Level II = Advanced Beginner
- ❐ Level III = Competent
- ❐ Level IV = Proficient
- ❐ Level V = Expert

STEP 4: SELECT A HEALTHCARE TERRITORY

Identify an employment option you would like to target by analyzing and reviewing the traditional and emerging territories along the continuum of care discussed in Chapter 11, "The Market Research Department of *You, Inc.*"

Identify the geographical location most attractive to you as well as those locations that most likely contain your target market. Determine what employment trends or predictions might affect your choice. For example, if you are an infection control nurse, you might be interested in and qualified for the new homeland security roles related to bioterrorism.

Identify who your "customer," is; which employer is most likely to want what you have to offer? For example, the customer of the new B.S.N. graduate who wants to work in critical care but has no experience will find customers/employers in an acute care hospital that has its own on-site critical care training programs to develop the staff they can't find in the healthcare marketplace.

Complete the following:

Your target market is: _____

Your customer is: _____

Related societal and cultural trends are: _____

_____

Related employment trends are: _____

_____

Qualifications for this target market are: _____

_____

Are you currently qualified?
     ❏ Yes
     ❏ No
     ❏ Perhaps, if . . .

If you answered "no" or "perhaps, if ...": Select another option or develop a plan to qualify for this position; see Step 6.

STEP 5: KNOW HOW TO STAND OUT!

No business owner who intends to succeed would ever think of investing time, money, and other resources in a service or product without an awareness of who else was doing it and how they matched up against them. Neither should you! The way to keep your career satisfying and invigorating is to stand out so you don't fade out!

Answer the following questions:

How is your product/service (your nursing skills and competencies) as good or better than that of others who have the same or similar skills and competencies? (Consider your experience, credentials, ongoing continuing education, professional certification, etc.)

_____

If you and ten other nurses applied for the job you want, what would make you at least as qualified, or even more qualified? (Consider transferable skills, interpersonal style, communications skills, etc.)

_____

In what ways would you improve the quality of service for the organization in which you are considering employment, beyond the minimum requirement of showing up for work and performing the tasks required in your job description? (Consider committees you have served on, interests you have such as diabetic teaching using Internet resources, etc.)

_____

How Well Do You Stand Out?

Review the lists of "Professional Experiences" and "Personal Characteristics" that follow. Using the following scale, rate each statement by placing a number in the space preceding the statement.

    1 = unable to compete effectively

    2 = need work to compete effectively

    3 = able to compete under some circumstances

    4 = able to compete fairly well, in most circumstances

    5 = able to compete effectively

Professional Experience

_____ Targeted, progressive, cumulative work as a generalist and/or specialist

_____ Has examples of work experiences that contributed value to the workplace

_____ Aware of, able to support, and can contribute to patient-focused care in a consumer-oriented business environment

_____ Diverse, transferable skills

_____ Cross-training

_____ Continuing education

_____ Computer literate and Internet savvy

_____ Bachelor of Science in Nursing

_____ Advanced educational preparation commensurate with career goals

_____ ANCC board-certification as a generalist or specialist (or other professional certification)

_____ Professional membership

_____ Additional: _____

Personal Characteristics

_____ Flexible, adaptive, assertive, confident, empowered

_____ Self-directed and team savvy

_____ Innovative problem solver

_____ Does not accept status quo

_____ Willing to take risks

_____ Learns from mistakes

_____ Conflict resolver

_____ Critical thinker

_____ Master networker

_____ Additional: _____

Note: This is by no means a complete list. It provides some examples that contribute to effective professional practice and employment in a fluid healthcare marketplace. Feel free to add to this list, personalizing it to your situation.

STEP 6: IDENTIFY NEEDS AND RESOURCES

Identify the professional, personal and interpersonal skills, resources, strengths, and abilities that are necessary to achieve your goal, namely, to look qualified to a potential employer. Include the potential obstacles and competing priorities that might exist. Fill in the blanks on the pages that follow:

Your Needs and Resources

Current, transferable skills (include non-nursing work)

_____

_____

Professional and personal strengths and weaknesses ("selling" points and areas needing improvement)

_____

_____

Your Needs and Resources (cont.)

Priorities (consider personal and professional situations)

_____

_____

Potential obstacles (personal and professional)

_____

_____

Inner barriers (limiting beliefs such as "I'm too old, too young, too busy")

_____

_____

Outer obstacles (such as lack of experience or credentials)

_____

_____

Training and education needs

_____

_____

Insurance, licensure, certification needs and issues

_____

_____

Your Needs and Resources (cont.)

Networking needs (see Chapter 13, "The Networking Department of *You, Inc.*")

_____

_____

Professional network: list key names

_____

_____

Personal network: list key names

_____

_____

Networking activities and events to target for attending

_____

_____

Financial needs and issues

_____

_____

Stress management and self-care needs

_____

_____

Your Needs and Resources (cont.)

Career support needed

_____

_____

Additional issues and considerations

_____

_____

Status of your "advertising" tools, "sales" skills, and professional network:

Resume

    ❐ Nonexistent

    ❐ Needs revision

    ❐ Updated and ready

Professional Portfolio

    ❐ Nonexistent

    ❐ Needs revision

    ❐ Updated and ready

Business Card

    ❐ Nonexistent

    ❐ Needs revision

    ❐ Updated and ready

Professional Network

    ❐ Nonexistent

    ❐ Needs revision

    ❐ Updated and ready

Your Needs and Resources (cont.)

Online Professional Network

❑ Nonexistent

❑ Needs revision

❑ Updated and ready

Sales/Interview Skills

❑ Nonexistent

❑ Needs revision

❑ Updated and ready

STEP 7: DETERMINE YOUR RISK POTENTIAL AND RISK TOLERANCE

How risky is the career goal you are contemplating, whether it's finding a new job or staying put for a while, returning to school or not, moving to another state this year or waiting until next year? These are big decisions and contain pros and cons, adding up to how much risk (if any) is involved in your decision. Reflecting on and identifying the risks entailed in your career goal helps you to decide what to do and when.

Profit and Loss Analysis

This term is used by business owners to denote a method of assessing overall financial risk. Here it is translated to mean the overall risk to be found in your selected career step, after weighing all the pros and cons.

Pros of following this career goal (reasons to pursue): _____

_____

Cons of following this career goal (reasons not to pursue): _____

_____

How I will profit from this career step is: _____

_____

What I might lose is: _____

_____

To determine how tolerable the risk is, consider how you completed the preceeding statements as well as the Risk Safety Assessment below, rating them according to the scale that accompanies it:

Risk-Safety Assessment

Read each statement below and rate it by placing a number in the space that precedes the statement according to the following scale:

1 = very safe	5 = more risky than safe
2 = mostly safe	6 = somewhat risky
3 = somewhat safe	7 = mostly risky
4 = more safe than risky	8 = very risky

_____ Personal or professional financial costs

_____ Influence of career goal on other priorities

_____ Ability to manage the stress of change

_____ Relative stability of the market you are targeting

_____ Additional personal or professional considerations: _____

_____

To interpret your score, total the points in the column preceding the statements and write it here: _____

Low risk   =   5 to 12 points

Moderate risk = 13 to 28 points

High risk*   = 29 to 40 points

High risk is a relative term and is actually a state that is pursued in order to obtain high benefits. The saying "nothing ventured, nothing gained" describes why risk is necessary for achieving goals. What is more important than the risk itself is your awareness of its presence and your preparation for it, hence the phrase, "calculated risk." Low risk situations may feel safe in the short run, but may not produce the kind of change and accompanying internal alertness necessary for personal and professional growth and development.

Is this career goal feasible?

☐ Yes

☐ No (rethink what you need to do)

☐ Perhaps, if I _____

STEP 8: CREATE A PLAN FOR YOUR GOAL

Begin by stating a clear goal, in specific and concrete terms. The more specific you are, the easier it will be to make it happen. Use action verbs and outcomes that can be measured or seen. For example, *"I will find a job as a nurse"* is vague and not easily measured. An example of a goal that is stated in a way that will be more useful in tracking your progress is:

> Within two months, I will find a job as a medical-surgical nurse in an acute care hospital that has at least 500 beds and an orientation program of not less than two weeks.

State your goal here: _____

_____

Tasks and Target Dates

Now, identify the tasks you need to do in order to achieve your goal. For example, this may include updating your resume, among other things. Again, make the task as specific as possible, breaking it into its smallest components. The process of getting a resume written or revised may have many steps associated with it, such as finding your old resume, talking to colleagues about their resumes, or making an appointment with a resume writer. Each task should have a target date of completion to keep you on track. Use the Marketing Plan on the next page to organize the goals and tasks required to achieve your goal.

Evaluation and Revisions

It is often necessary to revise your goals. This may not be evident until action is taken and you have an opportunity to evaluate the results. Keeping track of your progress in this way helps you make the revisions that are essential to achieving your goal. For example, as you move along, it may become clear that the goal of mounting a job search is totally mistimed and needs to be delayed for a while. Or, you may discover that the target dates were too ambitious and while the goal is still feasible, you need to adjust the task list and timeline to something more realistic.

Marketing Plan

	Tasks	Target Dates	Outcomes	Revisions
	(What actions are needed?)	(By when?)	(Evaluate the results and identify what's next)	(Develop new goals and/or tasks as needed)
Goal 1				
Goal 2				
Goal 3				

STEP 9: JOB SEARCH STRATEGIES

Now that you have a marketing plan for what you plan to achieve, a new job for example, it's time to determine where to take it, who might be interested, who your "customer" is.

The more *scheduled* time you are willing to devote to your job search, the more it will pay off for you. There is more to finding a new job than sending out a resume and then sitting back, waiting for the phone to ring. Some tips to keep you on track are:

- Keep track of your progress, in writing, by using the Marketing Plan you completed on the previous page.

- Set aside scheduled time each day to track your progress.

- Create a space in your home to keep related supplies and information. Consider including some motivational or inspirational material in the form of quotes, pictures, or symbols to encourage you.

- Start a folder or develop a filing system for each employer contact you have made and note the time of the next contact, the result of the contact, your impressions of the conversation, and what the next step is.

- Think twice before sending out resumes and query letters to potential employers who may not be looking for what you have to offer. This kind of "shotgun" approach can disperse your energy, especially if time is short. Each letter you send requires follow-up contact of some sort, making this a very time-intensive way to search for a job. On the other hand, the payoff could be big if you are seeking a job that is not often advertised or is otherwise hard to find.

- Tell everyone in your professional and personal network (online and in person) what kind of job you are seeking.

- Use the job postings within your present organization to generate "leads" and possibilities; ask your peers and colleagues in other organizations to do likewise for you.

- Attend job fairs. Don't forget your resume, dress professionally, and expect to be interviewed by potential employers.

- Peruse healthcare and nursing-specific classified ads in newspapers and nursing publications such as *Advance for Nurses* and *Nursing Spectrum*. It is a good idea to track job openings even if you are not considering making a move. This is an excellent way to monitor the current marketplace and keep your qualifications aligned with what employers are seeking in their potential employees.
- Use the Internet for employment information and job listings. Most healthcare organizations and institutions have home pages that not only describe them but have job postings as well. There are many nursing-specific career sites with job postings. Examples are:

  monster.com

  nursingspectrum.com

  www.advancefornurses.com
- Watch for "virtual job fairs," a new online recruitment strategy.

Networking is one of the best job search methods and is explored in the following chapter.

13

The Networking Department of *You, Inc.*

Networks are loose, dynamic webs of personal and professional alliances, forged for the purpose of obtaining knowledge, exchanging information, and sharing support. Networks are everywhere people are. And, in this new millennium, that means the traditional, in-person networks and the increasingly essential virtual networks of the Internet.

Networks can spontaneously emerge or can be intentionally created. You can take them with you, leave them behind, form new ones, merge old and new networks, or create formal or informal ones. Professional networks are essential to encouraging your *vision,* strengthening your *mission* and validating your *values/needs,* the three important components of your nursing product/service, all of which are necessary to ensuring career stability and satisfaction, especially during times of change. Refer to Chapter 10, "The Product Development Department of *You, Inc.*," for a full discussion of the meaning and importance of this to *You, Inc.*

In this age of information, the currency of exchange is knowledge and communication. The relationships in networks provide a way to obtain and utilize this currency, give it to others, and make it grow. Participating in networks is a way to invest in yourself and in *You, Inc.* that is as important as any financial investment you could ever make. Because registered nurses are knowledge workers, networks become essential links to and repositories for the vast amounts of ever-increasing information that you alone could never completely acquire or keep current enough. Twenty-first-century nurses know how to access the information they need, often rather quickly, from online networks and Internet portals, as well as from the many traditional in-person networks they keep active. Networks are information storehouses waiting for a time when you need what's in them.

Part of the satisfaction in networking is the opportunity to give to others as well as receive from them. It feels good to be on a listserv (online bulletin boards where you obtain information by asking/posting questions), see a message posted there by a new graduate in despair, and post a supportive response to him or her based on the experience you once had. The process of helping this new nurse provides you with an opportunity to experience your own growth, to see how far you have come. In fact, if all you do in a network is ask and take, the giving from others will eventually be harder to come by. Getting through the challenges of the nursing shortage will be easier with support and mentoring, a good deal of which can be done in networks and online.

A network represents the connections between and among people; some with direct relationships to each other, and others like distant relatives that are "once or twice removed." You may not know the person who has the information you need, but in a large enough network you are only "one or two degrees of separation" from obtaining it.

A NETWORK IN ACTION

Joan, a medical-surgical nurse with a B.S.N. and four years of experience on an oncology unit, is considering getting her board certification in oncology nursing at the generalist level. She wonders if this would really benefit her, especially since she is about to enter a master's program and is concerned about whether she will be able to do both at this time. She asks three people she works with, Tom, Mary, and Barbara, as well as Judy, a nurse in her electronic network, what they know about it. As you can see from the diagram on the following page, Joan got the information she needed through direct and indirect links. She communicated directly with only Tom, Mary, Barbara, and Judy, who each asked one person (Jill, Bob, Richard, and Marie), all of whom asked four people they knew (Donna, Larry, Joann, and Matt). Joan got the information she needed and then some, by extending her reach beyond those people she had direct contact with. When she found out that the certification exam would be given again next year, she felt less pressured about studying for it at the same time as beginning school in the fall. This information was quickly obtained from someone she didn't know as a result of her commitment to networking.

Joan's Network

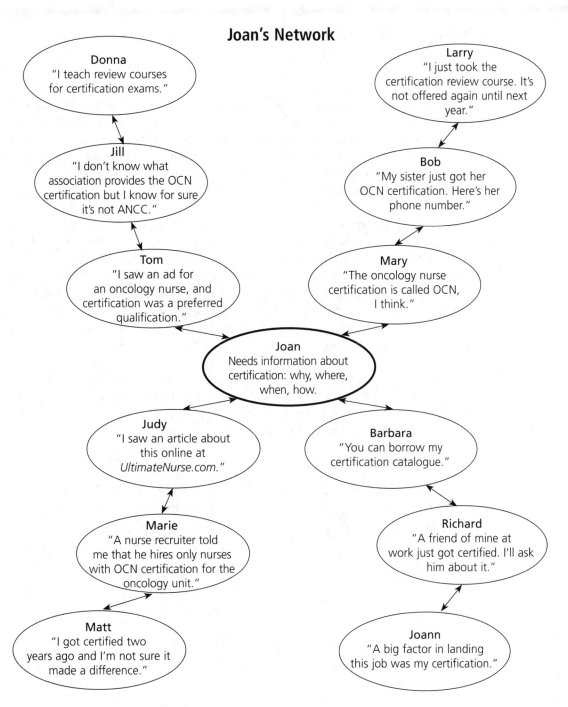

ONLINE NETWORKING

Listservs

Listservs are mailing lists, a kind of electronic bulletin board, often described as similar to a telephone "party line" but using email instead. Special interest groups such as universities, associations, and professional organizations maintain listservs in which you can post messages, ask questions, give answers, and track happenings. You can choose to just read what everyone is saying or jump in with your opinion by posting a response, to which someone else is likely to respond.

Many listservs are national and international, making the networking and relationship possibilities extensive. It is necessary to subscribe by contacting the listserv in which you are interested and following the directions they provide. Take into consideration that some listservs are very active, resulting in a significant amount of email. Many nurses (perhaps you were one of them) tracked the September 11th attack by means of listservs. It became a way to participate without being there, to share in the experience, to receive and get support, and to hear from and rally behind New York nurses and those from other states who were directly involved in the efforts to help.

The website of the American Nurses Association *(nursingworld.org)* has an excellent description of the use of listservs in nursing along with lists you can explore and subscribe to. They also provide a search engine for finding listservs of particular interest to you. Some examples of listservs are:

Case Managers	*Casemgr@cue.com*
Connecticut Nurses	*Listserv@uconnvm.uconn.edu*
NurseNet	*Listserv@listserv.utoronto.ca*
Breast Cancer	*majordomo@redbank.net*
Heart Talk	*Listserv@maelstrom.stjohns.edu*
Telehealth	*Listserv@maelstrom.stjohns.edu*

Usenet Newsgroups

These sites provide information relevant to a specific interest you may have in nursing or in healthcare, or a personal interest as well. Using newsgroups is an excellent way to keep current by using online rather than print resources. Summaries and bulletins arrive via email, usually in a newsletter-type format. The American Nurses Association *(nursingworld.org)* provides information about the use of newsgroups as well as listings. They provide direct links to the newsgroups they list as well as a way to search for ones of interest to you. Some examples are:

- Nurse Practitioner News Group
- Nursing Questions and Discussion
- Student Nurse Newsgroup

Email (Electronic Mail)

Using email makes it possible to establish and maintain relationships with nursing and healthcare colleagues, even for those with the busiest of lives, since staying in touch can be done from the comfort of your own home, or the place of your choosing, and at the time of your own convenience. Portable technologies such as telephones and PDAs make sending and receiving email something you can fit into your other activities with ease. The downside, of course is the stress of being overconnected. Refer to the self-care strategy called "know your limits" in Chapter 16 for a wider discussion of this 21st-century hazard.

THE BENEFITS OF PARTICIPATING IN NETWORKS

Personal and professional networks, whether traditional and in-person, or electronic via email, and listservs can benefit you in the ways described on the following pages. Next to each benefit or use of networking is a traditional, in-person example and an electronic-Internet example. Space is also provided for you to include your examples. An extensive list of Internet resources is also provided at the back of the book.

PROFESSIONAL NEED	TRADITIONAL NETWORKING EXAMPLE	INTERNET NETWORKING EXAMPLE
Track professional trends	Attend your annual state nurses association convention	Check the ANA website weekly *nursingworld.org*
Find coaches and mentors	Look around for possibilities within your current place of employment	Join at least three nursing listservs; ask directly for coaches or develop relationships with nurses online that can lead to this kind of relationship
Receive and give support, feedback, and encouragement	Schedule regular meetings with colleagues to provide opportunities for this	Schedule at least one "live chat" per week with nursing colleagues you work with or know from a listserv
Earn continuing education credits	Attend seminars and workshops on your days off and/or take advantage of what is offered in your place of employment	Investigate the many online distance learning sites with a wide range of topics
Search for employment opportunities	Call and/or tell everyone you know what kind of position you are looking for	Explore the websites of organizations in which you are interested to determine if there are openings; post a message on a listserv asking for information and the experience of anyone who worked there

PROFESSIONAL NEED	TRADITIONAL NETWORKING EXAMPLE	INTERNET NETWORKING EXAMPLE
Find the answer to a question about a procedure or technique about which you are unfamiliar and to which you are assigned the next day	Call your nurse friends and colleagues; find your preceptor before you go home for the day	Post a question on one of listservs; email your new nurse colleague in Alabama and ask him
Participate in job fairs	Schedule a day off and attend the job fairs you see advertised in the newspapers or in nursing publications	Watch for virtual job fairs conducted online by employers, (they are advertised in print publications and online); be prepared to submit your electronic resume and to be interviewed, or at least screened, as in traditional job fairs
Submit your resume	Hand resume out in person to colleagues or at a job fair	Submit an electronic version of your resume online (see Chapter 14 for how these differ from traditional ones)

PLACES TO LOOK FOR NETWORKING OPPORTUNITIES

Wherever there are people, you will find networks that are already established or people interested and available for new ones. A partial list of places follows. Write the places you have found networks in the column provided.

PLACES WHERE NETWORKS EXIST   **YOUR LIST OF PLACES**

Work relationships, present and former

School relationships, present and former

Professional associations

Conventions, seminars, conferences

Relationships with your own healthcare providers

Friends and neighbors

Health and sports clubs; social clubs

NETWORKING SKILLS AND STRATEGIES

Give *and* Get

Networks are established to meet the needs of *both* people, in a reciprocal way, over a period of time. What and how much you get from others when you need it will be determined by what you give or have previously given. While the computer term "garbage in, garbage out" may be a bit graphic as an example, it does convey the message. Pay attention to being a reciprocal partner in these relationships and you will benefit enormously.

Create Time for Networking

Challenge your belief that there is no time in your busy life for networking. Electronic networking, with its access to people and information at your convenience, has abolished that excuse. If for some reason you do not own a computer or have access to the Internet, make this a professional priority. If you are technologically phobic and have decided that you are going to get by without this essential 21st-century tool, the following statement from Chapter 4 is repeated here for your benefit: *"In your nursing practice, while you may be able to choose low-tech vs high-tech work, there is no longer any such thing as 'no-tech.'"* Utilizing the Internet is as relevant to your professional development as it is to the clinical work you do.

Be Proactive and Assertive

Take the initiative to establish conversations rather than always waiting to be approached. If this is not your strength, use networking opportunities to learn and develop it, practicing as you would any skill you were intent on learning. Consider seeking out a mentor or coach for assistance. Read a book. Talk to people online who have conquered this fear and are now comfortable approaching others.

Present Yourself with Confidence

Create and rehearse a brief introduction of who you are, a summary of your professional experience and/or personal interests. Consider an achievement of yours that others would be interested in, especially if it is relevant to the topic of the networking event you are attending. In addition, take care about the image you are presenting to others as revealed in your manner of dress, your attitude, your speech and grammar, and so on.

Formalize the Networking Experience

While networks can be formal or informal professional or social links, your approach to the process of networking should be formalized in that it is purposeful, organized, and focused on a purpose or goal you have set for yourself. The more structure you create around your networking experience, the more you will get out if it. Ways to formalize networking include:

- Conduct research to investigate which networks would best serve your needs.
- Participate in a variety of networks that represent your professional and personal interests, both traditional and electronic.

- Bring along your business card (you do have one, don't you?) to exchange with others. It creates an impressive image, and is also a way to keep track of who you meet and who you want to contact again. Chapter 14 contains information about business cards that you will find helpful. Establish a card file, traditional and/or electronic, to use when needed.

Increase Your Visibility

Attend meetings, join organizations, volunteer, and/or work on committees. Remember that networking is a mutual experience. Don't go to events just to see what may be in it for you.

Make Networks Work for You

When necessary, work at shaping the experience to meet your needs rather than complaining that the event you're attending or networking in general doesn't work for you. If this kind of proactive approach doesn't work, you may be in the wrong network; move on to others.

Practice Active Listening

Because networking is about mutuality, be a good listener, not just a talker. Try listening as this anonymous quote reminds us: *"Because God gave us two ears and one mouth, we should listen twice as much as we speak!"*

Consider Everyone You Meet a Contact

See the world anew, as a vast pool of networking possibilities, professional as well as personal. Then, smile, strike up a conversation, and look for opportunities to give and get information and support.

Smile, Smile, Smile!

It really does make a difference. You will look more approachable, and therefore, be approached more by others, which will make you feel good and result in making you smile even more! But, you need to start this feedback loop by smiling.

Open Windows When Doors Close

Work on transforming rejection or defeat into potential opportunities whenever possible. For example, if a nurse recruiter closed the door on you, so to speak, by not hiring you for the position you wanted, try opening a window of opportunity instead. Keep in touch with her, perhaps by sending her updated resumes periodically. Or, consider striking up conversations with her at professional meetings you may be at together. In this way, she becomes a link in your network, a possible connection to other work opportunities.

Trust the Process

Make networking an adventure by trusting that the links and connections in them can eventually lead to opportunities that you may not be able to identify at first. Be optimistic by believing in a positive result. Keep the process going by attending meetings and nurturing relationships.

CHAPTER 14

The Advertising Department of *You, Inc.*: Your Resume

WRITING YOUR RESUME

A resume advertises the nature of your nursing "business," what your self-owned nursing practice, *You, Inc.* has to offer. It creates the opportunities for dialogues with potential employers/purchasers of your nursing skills and competencies. A resume is an advertisement that may not directly get you a job, but like all advertisements will call attention to what you have to "sell." A well-written resume opens the door to the interview that is really a sales process and will be discussed in the following chapter.

A resume is a work in progress, an externalized representation of your professional nursing identity. As such, its style and content will grow and change over time, just as you do. There is a reassuring autobiographical quality to a well-written resume that becomes almost like a mirror, reflecting where you have been and what you have done while pointing the way to what you may do in the future. While employers may "own" your job and make decisions about its design and longevity, your resume represents what you own; namely, your work, your achievements, and your experiences. It represents what belongs to you after leaving the particular work environment in which work experiences occurred.

To keep your resume up-to-date and ready for your next career move, review and update it approximately every six months since futurists and forecasters say that significant changes affecting how you live and work are expected to occur with that frequency. This will give you a degree of reassuring control and preparedness during the constant change and permanent transition typical of today's healthcare workplace.

A resume is a summary of your experience and achievements, worded in short phrases. It is not a job description. It is not a complete description of everything you've done. In fact, a well-written resume should create some questions—but not confusion—in the reader's mind, questions that could be asked of you in the interview. This gives you the opportunity to "sell," to convince the employer that you have the nursing skills, competencies, and experiences that he or she needs. It allows you to emphasize the match between the employer and your abilities, and perhaps most important, to use the reactions of the interviewer to further shape your responses.

Periodically revising your resume is a way to align and realign your professional identity, a way to remind yourself of where you've been and what your best experiences are. The process of writing a resume is likely to rescue from memory skills and achievements previously overlooked. Revisions also give you the opportunity to rephrase and therefore realign your skills with current marketplace needs, thereby making you more employable. Many such realignments can be expected throughout your nursing career, and in fact, are a sign of a well-worn career path.

An excellent way to write or revise your resume is to create it with someone who can provide feedback and objectivity and help you shape it into the best possible sales tool. Consider working with a friend or colleague who has good writing skills and who can be objective about you. If you decide to use a professional resume writer or career coach, be sure you are involved in co-creating it. Allowing someone else to produce the resume in your absence denies you a level of involvement that serves to increase your confidence in *You, Inc.*, in the professional identity that your resume represents. If you choose to work on it alone, consider showing it to others for feedback.

Potential employers will be looking for a match between your credentials and experience on one hand and the requirements of the job needing to be filled on the other. Choose your words carefully and economically. Too many words, repetitions, or irrelevant data will work against you and may even eliminate you from the pool of people being considered.

RESUME APPEARANCE

Your resume should be typed in a font typically used in business and professional documents such as Times Roman or Arial. The size of the font should be 11 or 12 points. Avoid frilly, decorative fonts and use bolding, italics, and bullets sparingly.

Pay close attention to any special instructions requested by potential employers who plan to scan your resume into a computer. Since the computer cannot accurately scan anything decorative such as bullets or fancy fonts, ignoring these instructions may eliminate you from consideration. Generally, this is also true for resumes that are submitted online.

The resume can be one to two pages in length, but never more than two. Set the margins of the paper so that the information can fill the page with enough white space (empty space surrounding the typed words) to make for easy reading. Absence of white space indicates an attempt to cram too much material into too small a space, and for this reason a two-page resume, when necessary, is advisable.

Use professional stationery with matching envelopes in white or off-white. It's acceptable to neatly handwrite the address on the envelope; in fact, a handwritten envelope may indicate a personal but still professional touch.

Keep in mind that there is no one way to write a resume. After following the generally accepted guidelines presented here, it is a matter of personal preference. The type of resume described here is called the reverse chronological resume, in which the most recent professional experience appears first. An alternative is the skill-based resume, or some combination of both. Consult the print and online resources at the back of the book for more information about writing your resume. Most nursing career and networking sites have resume information. Some also have listings of resume services as well as tutorials, for example the University of Minnesota *(umn.edu)*.

GUIDELINES FOR RESUME PREPARATION

1. Contact Information

Place your name, credentials, address, and phone number centered on the top of the page. A line that separates this identifying information from the remainder of the text provides a format style that makes reading easier and quicker. Whether you choose to punctuate the initials of your credentials is a matter of personal preference. While the standard across all professions is typically to punctuate, in nursing punctuation is often omitted. The following example presents an unpunctuated style, but many nurses do punctuate.

SALLY SMITH, BSN, RN
75 East Main Street, #7A
New York, NY 10010
(100) 100-1000
Cell phone: (917) 100-0000
Email: sallynurse19156@aol.com

2. Profile or Summary of Qualifications

Use this in place of a job objective, which tends to limit and perhaps pigeonhole you. A job objective can be included in the cover letter that accompanies each resume you send out. Guidelines for writing a cover letter are included at the end of this section.

You might wait until your resume is completed to write the profile so that you have a better sense of what you want to include. A profile is a summary, not a complete repetition of your resume. It should highlight your best "selling" features as well as the kind of characteristics that employers are looking for today.

Profile Examples

Here's an example of what a new graduate's profile might look like:

Resourceful Registered Nurse with healthcare experience as a certified emergency medical technician and a proven work history, ready to apply transferable skills, including first-aid and basic life support, and a lifelong interest in nursing. Excels in settings requiring independent decision-making as well as team collaboration. Excellent organizational and critical thinking skills.

This is what a more experienced nurse might write:

Highly motivated and resourceful Registered Nurse with demonstrated effectiveness in the managed care environment as well as solid medical-surgical experience in acute care and community settings. Proficient in communicating and facilitating the acceptance of controversial managed-care concepts. Excels in advocating for patients within this cost-sensitive environment. Capable of prioritizing multiple responsibilities in fast-paced environments.

3. Your Education and Credentials

If this section becomes too lengthy, consider including a portion of it after the description of your professional experience.

License and Certification

Identify the state(s) in which you are licensed. It is not necessary to include your license number. Instead, carry your license in your professional portfolio, described later in this chapter, and take it with you to the interview. Include professional board certification from the American Nurses Credentialing Center (ANCC) and other professional associations.

Education

Place in reverse chronological order, including if currently enrolled. This section is for your formal nursing education, undergraduate and graduate.

Continuing Education

An extremely important "selling" and balancing feature to compensate for gaps or deficiencies in formal education or experience.

Professional Affiliations and Membership

Another important "selling" and balancing feature, demonstrating professionalism and commitment.

Special Abilities

Include foreign languages spoken, sign language, computer and Internet skills, and any other special talents.

Awards and Honors

This is no time for modesty. If you've won any, say so.

Publications and Presentations

Mention any articles you may have written or any occasion where you were required to convey educational information to groups of people.

Examples of how these seven categories just discussed might look are on the following page.

Examples of Education and Credentials

License and Certification	Registered Professional Nurse, New York and New Jersey Certified Medical-Surgical Nurse, ANCC
Education	Bachelor of Science, Nursing, Adelphi University (in progress) AAS, Nursing, Salem Community College (1998)
Continuing Education	Basic Cardiac Life Support AACN Cardiology Education Update (2001) Case Management for staff nurses IV Certification
Professional Affiliations	American Association of Critical Care Nurses Sigma Theta Tau International Nursing Honor Society New York State Nurses Association
Special Abilities	Fluent in Spanish and sign language Beginning competence with computers, including Windows, word processing, and the Internet
Awards and Honors	Dean's List, Salem Community College (2000) Outstanding Academic Achievement Award, Salem Community College (1999) Listed in *Who's Who Among American College Students* (2001) Distinguished Nursing Practice Award, Circle Hospital Center (1999)
Publications and Presentations	Grand Rounds Presentations: Care of the Dying Patient, Brooklyn Hospital (2001) Nursing Grand Rounds: Mentoring of New Graduates, Brooklyn Hospital (1999). "Transition to Home Care for Acute Care Nurses," in *Advance for Nurses*, June 2001

4. Description of Your Experience

List your relevant jobs in reverse chronological order (meaning, your most recent experience appears first) in any of the following categories that apply:

- Professional nursing experience: for work as an R.N. or nursing student
- Additional healthcare experience: for jobs other than R.N., such as L.P.N., nursing assistant, and emergency medical technician
- Additional work experience: for work outside of healthcare
- Volunteer work experience: for unpaid experiences (highly recommended!)

Use action verbs such as *provided, taught, created*, and *supervised* in your descriptions (see list below). When describing work experiences outside of healthcare, identify and describe relevant transferable skills. Examples of transferable skills are: triage of accident victims as an emergency medical technician, or customer-service skills used when employed as a bank teller.

To create phrases for your resume, begin each entry with an action verb, and write the phrase in "telegram style" rather than in full sentences (see the "Professional Experience" examples). The list of action verbs that follows is divided into categories of job skills relevant to the descriptions you might be creating. Take a look at all the lists as the verbs can often be applied to more than one skill set.

Action Verbs

Communication Skills

clarified	communicated	conferred	defined
described	developed	explained	formulated
listened	lectured	referred	

Creative Skills

adapted	began	composed	conceptualized
created	designed	initiated	originated
performed	reshaped	revitalized	

Action Verbs (cont.)

Financial and Information Skills

accounted for	administered	appraised	assessed
budgeted	computed	forecasted	measured
planned	prepared	processed	projected

Helping Skills

advocated	assessed	assisted	cared for
coached	collaborated	contributed	diagnosed
educated	helped	provided	rehabilitated

Leadership Skills

achieved	assigned	completed	delegated
directed	expanded	headed	led
managed	pioneered	resolved	supervised

Management Skills

administered	coordinated	directed	established
improved	initiated	managed	organized
planned	produced	scheduled	supervised

Organizational Skills

charted	collected	distributed	executed
implemented	maintained	monitored	ordered
organized	prepared	provided	reviewed
scheduled			

People Skills

coordinated	collaborated	consulted	empowered
encouraged	facilitated	interacted	led
motivated	organized	participated	

Action Verbs (cont.)

Research Skills

analyzed	collected	compared	conducted
critiqued	detected	determined	diagnosed
evaluated	formulated	gathered	identified
interviewed	investigated	located	organized
researched	searched		

Teaching Skills

adapted	clarified	coached	developed
evaluated	facilitated	individualized	instructed
motivated	taught	trained	

Technical Skills

adapted	applied	converted	designed
developed	maintained	remodeled	restored
replaced	solved	specialized	utilized

Each description should include dates of employment, job title, and name and address of organization (city and state are sufficient; full address can appear on application, if necessary). Start each description of your work experience with a phrase that orients the reader to the size and nature of the agency for whom you worked, as well as the general scope of your responsibilities. Following this orienting phrase, create additional short and pithy phrases that describe your most important responsibilities and achievements. Avoid repetition if similar responsibilities occurred in more than one job.

Four samples of these descriptions of experience are:

Professional Experience: Example 1

7/91 to present *Clinical Office Coordinator, Bronx Oncology Associates, Bronx, NY*

- Provide nursing care and administrative support to a high volume, 19 RN, 8 M.D. practice for the diagnosis and cutting-edge treatment of cancer.
- Perform telephone triage, including intervention and referral.
- Conduct independent nursing assessments and develop plans of care in collaboration with physicians.
- Provide education, counseling, and emotional support to patients and families.
- Act as liaison between patient, physicians, and healthcare institutions.
- Coordinate inpatient, outpatient, and office services, including the monitoring of plans of care to ensure compliance with insurance reimbursement policies.

Professional Experience: Example 2

6/02 to present *Student Clinical Rotations, St. Joseph's School of Nursing, Staten Island, NY*

- Learned and practiced primary nursing care in collaboration with professional nursing staff and multidisciplinary team in a variety of clinical settings, including Med-Surg, ICU, CCU, ER, Pediatrics, Maternity, and Psychiatry.
- Developed, implemented, and revised written nursing care plans, including discharge planning.
- Provided teaching and emotional support to patients and families.

Professional Experience: Example 3

4/99 to 5/02   *Emergency Medical Technician, Brooklyn Emergency Medical Services, Brooklyn, NY*

- Provided prehospital emergency care, for sick and injured patients as part of a two-person ambulance response team.
- Provided intervention at the scene, including triage, treatment, transport to treating facility, and status report to receiving staff.
- Initiated and maintained advanced cardiac life support, including defibrilation at scene and during transport.
- Acted as preceptor to newly hired Emergency Medical Technicians.

Professional Experience: Example 4

3/00 to 9/02   *Staff Nurse, Mount Olive Medical Center, New York, NY*

- Provided primary nursing care to adults with complex medical-surgical illnesses, often requiring critical care interventions, on a 40-bed unit specializing in oncology, pain management, and hematological disorders.
- Proficient in a broad range of critical care skills such as hemodynamic monitoring, ventilator care, titration of cardiac medications, and advanced life support.
- Responsible for written nursing care plans, including assessment and intervention of rapidly changing patient status.
- Assigned to frequent charge responsibilities.

A completed resume might look like this:

SALLY SMITH, BSN, RN
75 East Main Street, #7A
New York, NY 10010
(100) 100-1000
Cell phone: (917) 100-0000
Email: sallynurse19156@aol.com

Profile:	Highly motivated and resourceful Registered Nurse with current experience and a proven track record in providing nursing care for the stable and critically ill adult and geriatric patient. Capable of managing multiple assignments simultaneously and efficiently. Excels in environments requiring independent decision-making and team collaboration. Able to interact effectively with management, staff, and patients from all levels and cultural backgrounds.
License	• Registered Professional Nurse, New York State License
Education	• Bachelor of Science, Nursing, The City College of New York, New York, NY (1986)
Continuing Education	• Basic CPR Certification • EKG and Cardiac Arrhythmias (1998) • IV Certification • Basic computer keyboard and Internet skills • HIV Nursing Care Strategies
Awards	• 1992 Nursing Employee of the Year, Oceanside Medical Center, New York, NY
Professional Memberships	• American Nurses Association, member • New York State Nurses Association, member
Additional Abilities	• Fluent in Spanish and sign language • Computer competence, including Windows, word processing, and the Internet

Professional Experience

7/94 to present	*Staff Nurse, Radiology Department, Mount Olive Medical Center, New York, NY* • Provide primary nursing care during a broad range of radiologic procedures to in-patients and out-patients of all ages with medical-surgical problems.

- Manage the nursing care needs of stable as well as critically ill patients during and while awaiting procedures.

- Assist during complex procedures such as MRIs and angiographies, including pre- and post-procedure assessment, and support of patient well-being during procedure.

- Administer oral contrast material; insert and monitor IV during administration of IV contrast.

- Assess and manage allergic and life-threatening responses to procedures.

- Provide patient and family teaching, including emotional support.

- Participate in quality assurance activities, including patient surveys and documentation.

2/89 to 7/94   *Staff Nurse, Intensive Care Unit, Oceanside Hospital, New York, NY*

- Provided primary nursing care to adult and geriatric high risk patients with complex medical and surgical needs on six-bed ICUs with a ratio of one R.N. to two to three patients.

- Responsible for written nursing care plans which included assessment and intervention of rapidly changing patient status, in collaboration with multidisciplinary team.

- Performed a broad range of critical care skills, including hemodynamic monitoring for patients with multisystem failure.

- Assigned to frequent charge responsibilities.

2/86 to 1/89   *Staff Nurse, Medicine, Highview Hospital, New York, NY*

- Provided primary nursing care to adult and geriatric patients with medical and neurological problems on a 26-bed acute care unit.

- Responsibilities included nursing care plans, including discharge planning; patient and family education, including emotional support; multidisciplinary collaboration.

- Assigned to frequent charge responsibilities.

COVER LETTERS

A cover letter needs to accompany the resume you give or send to prospective employers. A different cover letter should be written for each employment situation, rather than using a general letter to cover all circumstances. Once you customize one cover letter, it can be used as a kind of template, a model from which to create others. Yana Parker, in her book, *The Resume Pro*, suggests you think about the following questions to help you prepare your letter:

- Why do you want to work for that organization?
- What do you know about the organization?
- How did you hear about them?
- What do you know about the position you are applying for?
- How can you help that organization with its goals, i.e., what skills, competencies, and abilities do you have to offer?

Guidelines for a good cover letter, adapted from recommendations made by Parker, include:

- Address your letter to the person with the authority to hire you, or who has been designated to interview you for the position, i.e., the Nurse Recruiter or other administrator. When unable to obtain this information, use a functional title, such as "Dear Nurse Recruiter," not "To whom it may concern," or "Dear Sir or Madam."
- Show that you know a little about the organization.
- Phrase your letter so that it is professional, but still warm and friendly.
- Set yourself apart from the crowd. Try to find at least one thing about you, your skills, competencies, experiences, that is unique, and relevant to the position.
- Be specific. State the position you are applying for, and how you heard about the position.
- Be brief; a few short paragraphs, all on one page will suffice.[1]

An example of a cover letter is provided on the next page.

Sample Cover Letter

IRIS CARTER, B.S.N., R.N.
35 Blossom Way
New Paltz, NY 10000
(100) 100-1000
Cell phone: (999) 900-0000
Email: ICRN19156@aol.com

January 17, 2003

Jill North, R.N., M.A.
Director, Human Resources
New Paltz Hospital
7745 High Road
New Paltz, NY 12345

Dear Ms. North,
I would like to be considered for the position of psychiatric staff nurse in your acute admissions unit as you advertised in *The New York Times* on January 14, 2003.

I have a Bachelor of Science in Nursing with ANCC certification in adult psychiatric nursing at the generalist level. My most recent experience includes four years of psychiatric nursing experience in acute care as well as home care settings. Some of my accomplishments include:

- Participating in the opening of a new day care center for geriatric patients, including the orientation of newly hired nursing assistants
- Development of a standardized care plan for the confused patient
- Serving on the nursing shortage task force

Additional qualifications I can offer you are excellent communication and interpersonal skills, and the ability to work independently and in team-based settings.

The enclosed resume describes my experience and credentials in greater detail and I would welcome an opportunity to discuss it with you in person. I am available for an interview at your convenience.

I look forward to hearing from you.

Sincerely,

Iris Carter
Iris Carter, B.S.N., R.N.

FOLLOW-UP LETTERS

A follow-up letter is an opportunity to reinforce a positive perception of you. It is a professional way to maintain contact. Because the interview is not unlike a sales experience, the more contact you have with the person contemplating your services, and the more positive a perception they have of you, the more likely it is for you to make the sale, in this case, to land the job. Your follow-up letter should include the following components, adapted from Parker's *The Resume Pro*.

- A statement of appreciation to the interviewer for the opportunity to discuss the job opportunity
- A reference to something that was discussed as a reminder and reinforcement of your experience, skills, and so on.
- Additional information, or new reasons that you are interested in the job, perhaps based on what was discovered or exchanged in the interview
- An offer to provide additional information or participate in additional interviews conducted by others
- A clarification, when necessary, about something that was discussed in the interview, such as a question that was asked or an issue to which you want to add information
- An anticipation of hearing from them again, perhaps about a favorable outcome, or at least about the decision that will be made

See Chapter 15, "The Sales Department of *You, Inc.: Interview Skills*," for more discussion and a sample follow-up letter.

BUSINESS CARDS

Business cards are a relatively easy and inexpensive networking and sales tool that make an impressive professional statement that can set you apart from others. Carry them with you to exchange during seminars and networking events. End an interview with an assertive handshake, a warm smile, and a "leave-behind" in the form of a business card. Attach them to your resume to circulate at job fairs. A sample business card is on the next page.

Sample Business Card

Iris Carter, B.S.N., R.N.
Registered Professional Nurse

35 Blossom Way
New Paltz, NY 10000

Telephone:	(100) 100-1000
Cell Phone:	(999) 900-0000
Email:	ICRN19156@aol.com

CREATE A PROFESSIONAL PORTFOLIO

A professional portfolio is a representative sample, a collection of documents about who you are professionally and what you have to offer. It contains an accumulation of information related to your professional life; a kind of historical chronology of your activities. It's almost a kind of professional diary. It contains the documented elements and examples, such as copies of your credentials, diplomas, letters of reference and recommendation, of your professional identity, gathered into one portable package that can be carried to interviews.

Your portfolio can have a private and a public section. The private section can be used to safeguard and keep track of important professional documents, accounts of your nursing work life, such as your license, certification information, and continuing education dates. You select from the private section of your portfolio what would be most relevant at a job interview. The public section is what you want others to see about you and what you have to offer. It's a sales tool, like a marketing book used by salespeople to demonstrate their wares. It may be tailored for the occasion by supplementing it with material from the private section of your portfolio, as indicated, and should contain:

- Broadcast letter that introduces you
- Letters of reference and recommendation
- Typed list of three to six personal and professional references
- Your resume
- Business cards

- Copies of your professional credentials including
    Diplomas
    Transcripts
    Continuing education certificates
    Performance appraisals
- Samples of professional achievements and activities such as:
    Letters of commendation or recognition
    Articles you have published
    Participation in poster sessions
    Anything that documents your professional or personal accomplishments

Many nurses have long used a variation of this portfolio as a filing system to keep these professional documents safe, as well as accessible when needed. Today's business-savvy nurse takes this a step further and uses her portfolio as a sales tool, as a way to stand out from others. In addition, because 21st-century nurses will be moving around the healthcare workplace much more frequently than those in previous generations, your portfolio becomes an important traveling companion to chronicle your travels and keep the historical data about it organized. In some ways it may serve as a way to reminisce and recount, and then to feel proud about where you've been and what you've done. It can become the mobile equivalent of your own personnel file, similar to the one your employer keeps about you, serving to remind you of your accomplishments.

Your portfolio can be as creative and imaginative as you are and, in fact, is an actual demonstration to a potential employer about your creativity, confidence, and assertiveness. It becomes a selling feature in and of itself! Consider using a colorful binder with interesting dividers. Take care, however, that it doesn't get too information-intensive, complex, or overdone; keep it unique and professional.

15

The Sales Department of *You, Inc.*: Interview Skills

An interview is a sales experience in which the potential employer is your customer. In fact, the entire healthcare marketplace contains many potential customers to whom the Nurse CEOs of *You, Inc.* can consider "selling" the services of their self-owned nursing practice. Refer to Chapter 9 if you still need convincing that all nurses are self-employed, even if they work for others.

The interview is your opportunity to present your best features to a potential employer, which translates into your credentials, experiences, skills, and talents. Your challenge is to convince this employer, to "sell" them on the idea that you have what they need, that they should "buy" what you have to offer, namely your ability not only to do the job they are looking to fill, but to excel at it, and that even though they may be considering others, you're the one they should select.

Millie, a newly graduated nurse applying for her first job, provides an example of what selling can look like. She has just been interviewed for a position in the critical-care unit of a major medical center that will provide her with a 16-week training and internship program. This organization accepts only four candidates every six months and Millie knows that more than four people were interviewed. While she has been told that if she is not considered this time she can reapply in the future, she doesn't want to wait that long. Recalling the interview, she remembered the nurse manager of the critical-care unit telling her that he expects 100 percent from his staff, so she wrote a follow-up letter saying, "You said that you expected 100 percent from your staff, and I wanted you to know that you can count on 120 percent from me." She included samples of two teaching tools she had developed as a volunteer for a health fair in which she had participated during her senior year, along with a description of her demanding student schedule that included working part time as a nursing assistant.

Millie got the job. During the training program, the nurse manager told her how impressed he was by her persistence and motivation to pursue what she wanted. She had sold him on the idea that she should not be passed over.

THE INTERVIEW AS A SALES EXPERIENCE

If the image of the pushy car salesman or intrusive telemarketer interferes with your ability to "buy" the idea that you are "selling" during the interview process, consider a less stereotypical way to think about it so that you can benefit from this useful career strategy. Believe it or not, you already are a salesperson!

Selling is a natural part of all communication; in fact, sales pitches are inherent in almost all conversations. Every time you talk to someone about your point of view, every time you attempt to convince another person to do something they may feel unsure of, an element of sales is involved. In fact, right now I am trying to "sell" you on the idea that selling is something that you can do, should do, and actually already do. I want you to "buy" this concept. And, right now, you may be acting like a salesperson too, as you try to "sell" me on *your* point of view about it, perhaps that selling is incompatible with nursing practice.

If you still haven't bought the sales concept, or believe nurses don't/shouldn't "sell," consider this: teaching a new diabetic to give himself insulin injections when he is convinced that he will never be able to do so is a sales experience. Or, reassuring a new mother that she will indeed learn how to care for her first newborn is also selling. As is teaching sex education to adolescents and "selling" them on the need for protected sex.

The same element of persuasion that is involved in patient education or in much of your communication can be used on your own behalf in a job interview. Just as a sales person can be a helpful ally when you are purchasing something you need but don't completely understand, so can you be helpful to your employer in your mutual quest for a satisfying and productive employment relationship.

WHAT SALES PEOPLE HAVE TO TEACH US

At least 50 percent of the interview process takes place before you walk in the door. More accurately put, the interview is an appointment, sometimes brief, that is part of a bigger process and begins with the very first contact you have with the potential employer, whether it's the impression your cover letter and resume make, how you dress at a job fair, or your interaction with a receptionist on the phone. A good salesperson would use each of these opportunities to "close" the deal, to make the sale. There are actually a series of "closes" before, during, and after the interview itself that move you closer to or further away from your goal of landing the job.

"Closes" are like stages and each one is a minisuccess on the way to getting the job offer, which could be considered the final "close." The first close is whatever you had to do to get the interview, such as the quality of your cover letter and resume, how you interacted with the interviewer's secretary, and so on. Typically, a salesperson doesn't always begin by asking if you intend to buy something; he might first find out something about you, send you free samples, create opportunities for you to become curious about what he's selling, and then answer your questions about it, ask you if he can keep in touch, and so forth.

If you take the best of what salespeople have to offer, you have great guidelines for preparing and doing well in an interview. An example is to pursue the first "close," meaning, to do the follow-up work needed to sustain a potential employer's interest in your offer of the nursing skills and competencies you want to "sell" him, creating as many opportunities as possible to keep the sale alive. In the example at the beginning of this chapter, Millie did this by sending a letter following her interview, thereby continuing the dialogue and increasing her chances of making the sale of getting into the critical care training and internship program.

If you think this sounds too aggressive, think assertive instead and be sure to communicate in that way. Imitate what helpful salespeople do, not the telemarketer's intrusive communication style. Many books and seminars teach the sales process, which frequently includes how to deal with rejection. The fear of rejection, the concern that someone will turn you down or will not be interested in what you have to "sell," keeps some people/nurses from staying connected to the steps of selling or sometimes from trying to begin with. If this is true for you, understanding and adapting some of the major messages of the sales industry to your interview process can help you conquer this fear.

Major Messages from the Sales Industry

- Not everyone will be interested in your service or product.
- A percentage of people will buy it, perhaps ten percent (one in ten).
- This percentage can change depending on the fluctuations in the marketplace that decrease or increase interest. For example, the nursing shortage has increased the percentage of people/healthcare organizations currently interested in purchasing the services of nurses.
- If one in ten (ten percent) of the people will buy, that means it may take nine "nos" to get to one "yes." (This may be especially true in some areas of the healthcare marketplace, for example there will likely be less "nos" in acute care than in ambulatory care.)
- On average, the more "nos" you get, the closer you are to the eventual "yes" as long as you don't abort the process or give up trying.
- Even if someone is interested, that doesn't mean he or she will buy it that time.
- Because the potential to buy at a later date exists, staying in touch is essential to this future prospect and to building your professional network (as Millie did in the previous example).
- Objections to the purchase of your product/service may exist. Your challenge is to be ready for them, identify them when they occur, and then present information to overcome these objections. This does not mean overpowering or strong-arming people as pushy salespeople do but rather convincing the buyer to think differently. An example for nurses might be highlighting transferable skills to substitute for skills or experience not yet achieved. Anticipating these potential objections, which will come in the form of questions from the interviewer, will be discussed later in this chapter.

THE INTERVIEW PROCESS

The interview is not a single event but a series of tasks and experiences in a process that could be divided into three stages: preparing for the interview, the interview itself, and following up after the interview.

Test Your Interview Knowledge

Before reading further, test what you know about interviews by placing a check mark in the box preceding each statement below to indicate if you think the statement is true or false. The answers along with an explanation about each statement appear at the end of this chapter as a review.

1. ❐ True ❐ False   In order to appear natural and spontaneous, it is better not to prepare responses ahead of time.

2. ❐ True ❐ False   Be cautious about your body language because 40–50 percent of communication is nonverbal.

3. ❐ True ❐ False   It is important to maintain direct eye contact at all times with the interviewer.

4. ❐ True ❐ False   It is better to interrupt the interviewer than to forget to say or ask something.

5. ❐ True ❐ False   Referring to a list when asking questions gives the impression of being unprepared.

6. ❐ True ❐ False   Asking for a tour of the unit you may be working on appears intrusive.

7. ❐ True ❐ False   Asking about the next steps or what your chances are of getting the job is too aggressive.

8. ❐ True ❐ False   Writing a follow-up letter to the interview is redundant and a waste of the interviewer's time as well as yours.

9. ❐ True ❐ False   If you decide to take another position before you hear the results of the interview, it's better to withdraw your application without saying why.

10. ❐ True ❐ False   If you do not get the job, it is not a good idea to discuss the reasons why with the interviewer.

PREPARING FOR THE INTERVIEW

Learn about the Organization

The more you know about your potential employer, the better prepared you will be to do well in the interview, not only by responding well to the questions you will be asked, but by appearing knowledgeable about the organization as well. Ways to familiarize yourself with the organization include conducting informational interviews (described below), exploring its Internet website, seeking information through your personal or professional network, and determining if it has or is planning to seek Magnet status certification. Refer to Chapters 1 and 2 for discussions about how organizations with this certification provide optimal nursing practice environments.

Conduct Informational Interviews

An informational interview is not a casual chat with someone you just happen to meet but rather a planned experience in which you select one or more persons you hope will tell you about the position you are seeking, someone who is working in that organization or who has done the kind of work you want to be doing. It's a way to get the inside scoop.

The people you select to interview can be those you know, or those who are referred to you by others (use your network here!). You can also find candidates for your interview online in chat rooms or on one of the listservs to which you subscribe (you do belong to at least one listserv, don't you?).

To get the most out of informational interviewing, tell the people you plan to interview in advance the purpose of the meeting and what in particular you are interested in hearing about. This will give them the time they need to consider the most helpful responses for you. Prepare a list of questions that might include the following:

- Do you enjoy your work? Are you doing what you expected or wanted to do when you considered this job?
- What does a typical workday look like?
- Describe the communication and relationships you have with your coworkers, with managers, with physicians.
- How are disputes and conflicts handled?
- What advice would you give to someone considering working here?

Add your questions here:

_____

_____

_____

Determine If Your Qualifications Match the Employer's Needs

To prepare effectively for the interview, it is important that you know how closely your nursing skills, competencies, and experiences match what the employer is expecting. Once you know this, you can compensate for what might be missing. If, for example, your IV and phlebotomy skills are five years old (experience is often not considered current after three years), taking a refresher course before the interview will go a long way in reassuring the interviewer that you were aware of the need to update and took care of it by being proactive, rather than sliding by or thinking it would not be noticed. Taking this action presents you as a responsible professional and communicates indirectly that you can be counted on to do the right thing, definitely an asset to any organization.

Refamiliarize Yourself with Your Resume

After you determine how closely you meet the requirements of the position you are seeking, review your resume to pre-select what you want to highlight in the interview and to remind yourself what you might need to compensate for as well. This includes identifying what your transferable skills are and how you plan to weave them in to the interview at an opportune time.

For example, let's say you are applying for a position as a direct care nurse in a psychiatric inpatient unit but have no formal experience as a psychiatric nurse. Your last position was on a medical unit in which you cared for a large volume of geriatric patients, many with dementia and psychosis. Let's further imagine that you not only enjoyed working with this kind of patient but in addition, your peers and colleagues used you as a resource when these patients were assigned to them. Let's also add that you developed a standardized care plan for these patients that became the unit-standard. Can you identify the transferable skills that could compensate for your lack of formal experience in psychiatric nursing? List them here:

_____

_____

_____

Anticipate Questions and Prepare Responses

The amount of time spent considering questions you might be asked and planning how you intend to respond to them will greatly influence the degree of comfort you have in the actual interview, and of course, how well you do. Remember, at least 50 percent of the interview process happens before you walk in the door, and a good part of that percentage is spent right here.

What follows are samples of questions you might be asked, along with examples of weak, ineffective responses to avoid, and more effective responses that have a greater potential to "sell" you to the interviewer. It is unlikely that you will be asked all of these questions. Use them as a guide to prepare your own responses or as a kind of self-assessment that identifies your areas of strength or weakness. Use the Interview Preparation Worksheet later on in this chapter to develop your own prepared responses.

Anticipated question: **Why do you want to work here?**
Ineffective response: You have good benefits.
Effective Response: You have an excellent reputation for patient care, and I am ready for the challenges of an acute-care medical center.

Anticipated question: **What makes you qualified to work on this kind of neurology unit?**
Ineffective response: I'm a hard worker.
Effective Response: In my med-surg and community health rotations (in nursing school), I cared for many neurology patients. I liked the complexity of it and my clinical evaluations from that rotation were excellent.

Anticipated question: **What are your strengths?**
Ineffective response: I like people and people like me.
Effective response: I'm flexible and able to adapt quickly. I'm also a good organizer, and work well with others.

Anticipated question: **What continuing education have you recently participated in?**
Ineffective response: A lot of different courses. Sometimes I send in those AJN tests, you know, those articles.
Effective response: I've just completed ACLS. I'm presently enrolled in IV certification. I'm planning to take an advanced physical assessment course in two months.

Anticipated question: **Tell me about your experience.**
Ineffective response: I've had experience in a lot of different areas, as you can see on my resume. (Note: Yes, the interviewer can read your resume. However, he or she also wants to hear you talk about it, so this is an opportunity for you to shine. A good resume should inspire questions in the interviewer's mind, giving you an opportunity to add to it, clarify, and shape your responses for the position you are currently seeking.)
Effective response: While I don't yet have R.N. experience, I have three years of hospital-related experience as a unit clerk and nursing assistant. My clinical rotations provided experience in all aspects of nursing, especially neuro patients, since we did our med-surg rotation on neuro.

Anticipated question: **What do you want from this experience?**
Ineffective response: I want to work days and I need health insurance.
Effective response: An opportunity to develop professionally, to share my ideas and skills. I am seeking new professional challenges. I also want to use this experience to qualify for ANCC board certification in med-surg nursing.

Anticipated question:	**Why did you choose to become a nurse?**
Ineffective response:	I like to help people.
Effective response:	It's a profession that offers upward mobility, diverse challenges, and the kind of personal contact I've always enjoyed.

Anticipated question:	**Tell me what you like to do best in nursing.**
Ineffective answer:	Making people feel better.
Effective answer:	I'm a good teacher, especially when it involves something complex like insulin administration. I know how to explain complicated things simply and it's gratifying to experience people's response to it.

Anticipated question:	**How do you deal with conflicts on the job?**
Ineffective answer:	I never have conflicts. I get along with everyone.
Effective answer:	I suggest that we discuss the issue to clarify the problem and check for misinterpretations. Conflicts are a natural part of the job and communication is essential to working them out.

Anticipated question:	**If I were to call your former employer for a reference, what would she say about you?**
Ineffective answer:	She would say I'm a good worker.
Effective answer:	I believe she would tell you about my flexibility, especially when the hospital was downsized three years ago. There was a need for unit clerks to rotate to other units. While I did it to cooperate, I have to say that I gained a lot too. It helped me improve my communication skills since there was more contact with patients and family on the other units.

Anticipated question:	**What do you think is most important about being a nurse?**
Ineffective answer:	Never miss a day of work.
Effective answer:	I believe nurses help people to heal themselves by supporting and sustaining them physically, mentally, emotionally, and spiritually until they can do this for themselves.

Anticipated question:	**What are your work-related goals for the next five years?**
Ineffective answer:	I don't know. I may be planning a family.
Effective answer:	I would like to be ANCC-certified in med-surg nursing and then begin thinking about graduate school.
Anticipated question:	**Why should I hire you instead of other applicants?**
Ineffective answer:	I have a lot of experience.
Effective answer:	In addition to my familiarity with the hospital environment because of my work here as a unit clerk, I can offer you the same kind of commitment and flexibility that my last employer remarked about in my performance appraisal.
Anticipated question:	**Describe yourself.**
Ineffective answer:	I'm married, have two children, and work hard.
Effective answer:	I consider myself flexible and enthusiastic. I enjoy the fast-paced nature of acute care hospitals. I get along well with people of all backgrounds. I was recently inducted into Sigma Theta Tau (the international nursing honor society). I'm very proud of that.
Anticipated question:	**Why did you leave your former job?**
Ineffective answer:	I was bored.
Effective answer:	Overall, I liked my last job. However, I felt ready for the challenges of an acute care medical center like this one, especially because you specialize in oncology.
Anticipated question:	**Since you haven't worked in med-surg for some years, how well will you function here?**
Ineffective answer:	Once you've learned med-surg, you never forget it.
Effective answer:	I have kept up by taking online continuing education classes and recently completed a refresher course. I volunteer at a rehab center regularly. I've also kept up by reading *AJN* and going to professional conferences. In addition, I'm a fast learner and feel confident in my ability to do this job.

Anticipated question:	**Are you IV Certified?**
Ineffective answer:	No.
Effective answer:	No. However, I am currently pursuing certification and have experience in monitoring IVs and managing IV therapy.

Anticipated question:	**Have you ever managed a large clinic?**
Ineffective answer:	Not really.
Effective answer:	No, but I have successfully managed my brother's graphic design business. Some of my responsibilities were taking telephone orders and resolving customer problems and complaints. I also organized his telephone contacts and developed a filing system of his customers.

Anticipated question:	**Have you had experience in home visits?**
Ineffective answer:	Yes.
Effective answer:	Yes, during my nursing school clinical rotation. I enjoyed it. I liked the increased autonomy and the more comprehensive assessments that were possible in home environments.

Questions You Should Ask

It is likely that you will be given an opportunity to ask questions at some point during the interview; typically this will be at the end. Should you think of questions as the interview is proceeding, inquire if you can ask them as they occur to you, or if you should wait until the end. It is always a good idea to ask questions. It demonstrates your professionalism and knowledge about important issues. Questions you could consider asking, especially if this information wasn't covered during the interview, follow. You might already know the answers to many of these questions, so it is not necessary or advisable to ask them all. Select the ones from this list that are most important to you.

- What is the role of the nurse in your organization? Or, what are the expectations of the nurse in this position? To whom would I be reporting?

- For organizations without Magnet status: Is your hospital planning to apply for Magnet status?

- For organizations with Magnet status: Has Magnet status changed the role of the nurse in any way?
- Can you tell me something about the relationships the nurses in this organization have with peers and colleagues?
- Can you tell me about your staffing ratios and staffing policies?
- How has your organization been affected by the nursing shortage? Is there anything specific you are doing about it?
- Can you describe your in-service education programs, especially for new roles and responsibilities?
- What are the opportunities for and policies about advancement in your organization?
- Can you tell me about the salary and benefits? (Always make this the last question unless the interviewer brings it up earlier.)

Questionable Questions

There are some questions that the law prohibits the interviewer asking you because they are discriminatory and not job-related. These questionable questions include anything related to your:

- Age
- Marital status
- Children or childcare needs
- Nationality
- Ethnicity
- Sexual preference
- Religion
- Financial status or credit issues

INTERVIEW PREPARATION WORKSHEET

Step 1 **Reflect on the job for which you are preparing to be interviewed and complete the following statements:**

List the qualifications the employer is seeking.

_____

_____

_____

Identify the qualifications you have.

_____

_____

_____

Identify the qualifications you don't have.

_____

_____

_____

Identify your transferable skills.

_____

_____

_____

Step 2 **After reviewing and re-familiarizing yourself with your resume and reflecting on your nursing skills and competencies:**

Identify your strengths (What you excel at, love doing, have gotten great feedback about, have experience in, etc.).

_____

_____

_____

Identify your weaknesses (What you are not good at, dislike doing, or have limited or no experience in, etc.).

_____

_____

_____

Step 3 **Identify how you plan to go about changing a weakness into a strength or how you will compensate for it.**

_____

_____

_____

Step 4 **Develop a prepared response for one of your weaknesses.**

_____

_____

_____

INTERVIEW PREPARATION WORKSHEET (CONT.)

Step 5 Develop a prepared response for one of your strengths.

_____

_____

_____

Step 6 Develop prepared responses for additional questions you anticipate being asked.

_____

_____

_____

THE INTERVIEW EXPERIENCE: TIPS AND STRATEGIES

It's natural to be nervous about being interviewed. The strategies that follow will help you manage your anxiety and harness that energy for productive use on your own behalf.

Arrive Early

Be compulsive about this. Arrive at least one hour prior to the time of the interview to allow for unexpected travel delays or difficulty in finding the interview location once you are inside the organization. Upon arrival, go directly to the interview location so that you know exactly where it is and then find a place nearby where you can sit quietly until the time of your appointment. Look for a place of worship, a coffee shop that is not too crowded, or a nearby park. You might also consider wandering around the block a few times if you are too restless to sit still.

Let Go and Rest/Relax

Utilize the same principle with which you are familiar (or should be!) when preparing for exams: at some point, you need to let go, stop studying, and get some rest, trusting that all the preparation you have done will allow the information you need to emerge spontaneously at the right time. Do this or any of the self-care strategies below, especially if you are anxious.

Self-Care Prior to the Interview

You may find one or more of the following strategies helpful:

- Get to bed early enough to feel rested on the day of the interview.
- Omit or decrease your intake of caffeinated beverages.
- Drink sufficient water to prevent dehydration from decreasing your energy or ability to think clearly.
- Breathe deeply enough, especially if you are anxious, to ensure the oxygenation is sufficient for thinking clearly.
- Eat breakfast, selecting foods known to give you high energy.
- Meditate, if this is a familiar technique to you.
- Visualize, seeing yourself successfully asking and answering questions, and then being offered the job.
- Use affirmations, saying something like, "I do well in interviews" or "I can interview successfully" or "I am qualified for this job."

Carry a Briefcase

A briefcase or other professional carry-all enhances your image and keeps you organized. It should contain additional copies of your resume, your list of references and recommendations to give the interviewer, paper and pen, your list of prepared questions, a small bottle of water in case you need it, and your professional portfolio (see Chapter 14 for a description of this important career tool).

Dress to Impress

Imagine the image you want to portray, and then dress accordingly. You've heard it all before:

- First impressions are lasting impressions
- A picture (your image) is worth a thousand words
- Actions (and in this case, appearance) speak louder than words

Don't let your appearance detract from the quality of the preparation you did for this interview or from the qualifications you bring. Dress like the professional you are. Just because you may wear scrubs to work, doesn't mean you should dress casually in the interview. Dress in a conservative manner. For women, this means a tailored suit or simple dress with a below-the-knee length, minimal jewelry, moderate makeup, stockings, low-heeled shoes, and a small handbag to accompany the briefcase in which you carry your professional portfolio. For men, a conservative suit and tie, white shirt, polished shoes, and your portfolio. Both women and men should omit perfume or cologne or at least keep it minimal.

Display Confidence and Respect

When escorted in to the office in which you will be interviewed, offer to shake hands (no limpness here!) and wait to be offered a seat. Greet the interviewer with minimal chatter and take your cues for responding from him or her.

Respond with Careful Thought

Keep your responses clear, direct, and succinct. Give enough information to answer the question but give careful thought to offering what is not being asked. Find the balance between too much and too little.

Ending the Interview

Thank the interviewer for the opportunity to be considered for the position, offer to shake hands again and (take a deep breath here!) ask what the chances are of your being hired. This assertive, proactive question gives you the information you need for the important follow-up phase of the interview process. Asked appropriately, this question also portrays you as confident and professional. You may be pleasantly surprised by hearing the intention to hire you (most likely following a check of your references) or at the very least what the next step in the process might be.

AFTER THE INTERVIEW

You're not done yet! There are two more very important steps to completing the interview process: the follow-up letter and a method for you to decide if you will accept the position if it is offered to you.

The Follow-Up Letter

Writing a follow-up letter is a professional response to an important professional experience and is well worth your time and effort. To begin with, it gives you an opportunity to strengthen weak responses by providing stronger ones after the interview when you are less anxious, as the following sample letter demonstrates. The letter will also reaffirm your interest in the position if this is the case, or at least thank the interviewer for the opportunity to be interviewed. The letter is likely to be kept on file along with your resume for a least one year, and may benefit you in the future.

A Sample Follow-Up Letter

Iris Carter, a new B.S.N. graduate, prepared for what she heard would be a very tough interview at an acute care hospital where she had her heart set on working. She knew (from the informational interviewing that she did) that she would be given a patient care scenario and asked to discuss how she would care for the patient. In the interview, the scenario she was given was the following:

"You are a nurse in the PACU (post-anesthesia care unit) and a patient who just had an abdominal hysterectomy is wheeled in from the OR. Give me two nursing diagnoses and two corresponding interventions for this patient."

Before proceeding, take this opportunity to imagine yourself responding to this question in an interview and write your response here:

_____

_____

_____

Iris's nursing diagnoses were related to the potential for bleeding and the potential for airway obstruction. After Iris offered several interventions for each diagnosis, she felt satisfied by her response. The interviewer appeared satisfied as well since she went on with the interview, as Iris later recalled.

When Iris reflected on the interview later, she realized she had forgotten one of the most important interventions of all, namely to check the patient's dressing for bleeding. Her initial panic subsided when she decided to include an explanation of this in the follow-up letter she planned to write. At first she considered ignoring the situation altogether, hoping the interviewer hadn't noticed, or that it wouldn't matter. She rejected this idea as wishful thinking and rightly decided that ignoring it might do more harm than good. The letter Iris wrote appears on the following page.

Iris Carter R.N., B.S.N.
35 Blossom Way
New Paltz NY
(100) 100-1000
Cell: (917) 555-5000
Email: CarterIris12345@juno.com

Jill North R.N., M.A.
Human Resources Department
New Paltz Hospital
7745 High Road
New Paltz, NY, 12345

January 12, 2003

Dear Ms. North,

Thank you for the opportunity to interview for the position of direct care nurse in one of the surgical units of your organization. I learned a lot about what you expect from your staff and feel sure that I will meet your expectations. I especially liked the tour you provided. It allowed me to see the action I was hoping for and increased my desire to be part of that team.

In thinking back to the question you asked about the patient with the abdominal hysterectomy, I realized I neglected to tell you that one of my interventions would be to check the patient's dressing for bleeding. This is definitely something I would know to do but somehow omitted because I was a little anxious in the interview. I would welcome an opportunity to respond to any other questions you might have about my ability to care for this type of patient. As we discussed in the interview, my clinical rotations in nursing school included the care of many post-operative patients and I have confidence in being able to care for them effectively.

I look forward to hearing from you.

Sincerely,

Iris Carter
Iris Carter

This letter says a lot about Iris's integrity and professionalism, a well as her sales ability. She portrays an image of someone who is concerned about quality patient care as well as someone who is willing to take responsibility and to learn from her mistakes. It would be hard to imagine an interviewer not being impressed by this kind of response, whether or not Iris was offered the position.

Employer Evaluation Checklist

This final step in the interview process will help you determine if the position for which you interviewed is indeed what you want to accept, should it be offered to you. Use the Employer Evaluation Checklist that follows to help you decide if a mutually satisfying match between you and the potential employer exists.

EMPLOYER EVALUATION CHECKLIST

Organization _____

Date of Interview_____

Contact Person _____

Place a check in the box provided to indicate your satisfaction with the employment potential of this organization. The more checks that appear, the greater the match between you and the employer.

- ❏ The institution bases its policies and procedures on specified nursing standards.
- ❏ The institution has Magnet status certification or is in the process of obtaining it.
- ❏ You will be reporting to a nursing manager and/or nursing administrator (in general this is preferred but not always necessary as long as there is access to nursing resources people should the need arise).
- ❏ The roles and responsibilities of the position were clearly and adequately explained (check this statement twice if the description was given to you in writing).
- ❏ The nurse-patient ratio was described and is reasonable; there is an approved administrative mechanism to negotiate a potentially unreasonable assignment.

❏ There are opportunities for administrative and/or clinical advancement.

❏ The orientation for newly hired staff is adequate; there is a preceptor program.

❏ There is continuing education and on-site training, especially for new roles and responsibilities; education is encouraged; some tuition reimbursement is provided.

❏ The starting salary for the position is satisfactory.

❏ The benefits package is satisfactory (health insurance, paid vacations, etc.).

❏ Specify additional factors of importance to you on the following lines:

_____

_____

_____

ANSWERS TO INTERVIEW QUIZ

The answers to the interview quiz earlier in this chapter appear below, accompanied by an explanation. Use this information as a review of the material in this chapter.

1. **False.**   Preparation is essential for successful interviewing. It also helps you to lower your anxiety and manage your stress.

2. **False.**   A whopping 90 to 95 percent of communication is nonverbal and takes the form of body language, manner of dress, tone of voice, attitude, and behaviors such as punctuality, assertiveness, and so on.

3. **False.**   No one maintains eye contact 100 percent of the time. Looking away periodically and briefly as you ponder the answers to questions is normal.

4. **False.**   A better option is to jot down notes about questions you have and wait for the best opportunity to ask them, perhaps at the end of the interview, or when asked if you have questions. However, flexibility is the key here. If you are confused, it's better to clarify this with a polite interruption rather than feel lost and unable to respond or continue.

5. **False**.   Just the opposite is true. Bringing a list makes you look prepared and interested enough to have given considered thought to the employment situation. It will also decrease your anxiety.

6. **False**.   This is an appropriate request. Taking a tour can provide a different and perhaps welcome source of data that words cannot completely convey.

7. **False**.   This is an assertive question that conveys confidence and professionalism. It is also an essential sales strategy for planning your follow-up and the focus of your efforts and energy. Assertiveness and productivity are essential characteristics of successful 21st-century nurses, and well worth strengthening your skills in.

8. **False**.   Not only does this kind of follow-up demonstrate that you know how to conduct yourself professionally, it also continues contact with the employer beyond the interview to keep your name familiar. In addition, it gives you the opportunity to strengthen weak responses caused by anxiety or insufficient preparation.

9. **False**.   A written letter expressing appreciation for the time and consideration granted you and a brief reason for your decision maintains the relationship and keeps the door open for future possibilities. It is a way to grow your network as well as your reputation.

10. **False**.   Asking this question could strengthen your approach for the next interview and may also keep the door open for the future should another job at that organization become available.

CHAPTER 16

The Resilient Nurse: Self-Care Strategies

All of us who are working as nurses today were born in the 20th century. While that is where we began this adventure called our life and, most likely made the decision to become a nurse, we have journeyed a distance from there and find ourselves living and working in the 21st century, a place where the experiences we take for granted today once lived only in the imaginations of futurists and science fiction writers. A place far more complex than just a few generations ago. A place where it is possible to carry around palm-sized (or smaller) devices for staying in touch with one another, (remember *Star Trek*?) untethered to wires for power that would otherwise restrict where we could go, how far we could travel, or how quickly we could get there.

> "In a fast-paced, continually-shifting environment, resilience to change is the single most important factor that distinguishes those who succeed from those who fail."
>
> –Daryl R. Conner in *Managing at the Speed of Change*[1]

Just as these wireless wonders of technology make our lives easier, so do they make them more complicated, demanding, and stressful by increasing the number of things to do, the speed at which they need to get done, and the number of people waiting for you to respond to their needs, requests, and demands, NOW! So, we invent a word to describe the skill needed to manage this and other wireless wonders of technology, namely *multitasking*, which becomes the only way to cope with the ever-growing number of things to do.

HIGH TECH, HIGH ANXIETY

This relentless activity and the speed that accompanies it is a reality of our nursing practice as well, accompanied by the added feature that the well-being of others is reliant on our ability to use a vast array of ubiquitous, often complicated, and ever-multiplying healthcare technologies. Simultaneously, we must assure that this "high tech" environment is also accompanied by "high touch," so that the essence of nursing, namely, caring, is not lost. Oh, and did I forget to mention that there are ever-fewer numbers of us to do this for an ever-growing number of sicker and sicker patients?

Whew!!!

The mental, emotional, and physical frenzy often created in response to the demands of this way of living and working require an attention to the conservation of our energy, to the preservation of our self more urgently needed than just a few short decades ago. While it is true that change has always been a feature of life, the volume, momentum, and complexity of change which characterize the early years of this new millennium are different, and captured well in the following passage by Daryl Conner in *Managing at the Speed of Change:*

> "Mark down the date that you read this book. I can say with great confidence that in three years you will look back on this period as 'the good old days' when life was relatively calm. Our world as it is now will look slow and uncomplicated compared to what it is sure to become within the next few years; you have more control and less ambiguity today than you are likely to have for the rest of your life."[1]

Just as the word *multitasking* was invented to describe what we have to do to cope with all the wireless (and wired) wonders in our life, so is there a phrase to describe the experience we have with this kind of change and what awaits us as a result: "permanent transition," meaning just as you adapt to something that's changed, just as you make the transition to something new, it is about to shift shapes, in a small or a big way, requiring you to shift along with it. (Think of the fast-evolving generations of computer programs, requiring update, after update, after update . . . !)

THE RIDDLE OF THE LILY PAD

To understand the enormity of this and therefore to grasp the impact this kind of change is having on your personal and professional lives, Conner asks you to consider the "Riddle of the Lily Pad":

> On day one, a large lake contains only a single, small lily pad. Each day the number of lily pads doubles, until on the 30th day the lake is totally choked with vegetation. On what day is the lake half full?

If your answer was the 29th day, you are right! It takes 29 days for the first half of the lake to fill with lily pads, but only one more day for the lake to become overwhelmed.

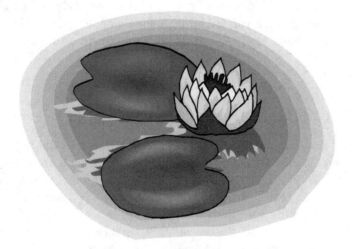

The lesson of the lily pad riddle is:

> Because you can't stop the lily pads (which represent change) from multiplying, you need to expand the lake's (your) capacity to absorb (cope with) it (change).

Stop, slow down, and reflect for a moment:

What would *expand your capacity* to meet the challenges of change, which paradoxically will continue to be the "permanent status quo" of your personal and professional life?

What will *strengthen your ability* to cope with stress, the twin partner of change, so that you don't collapse under the weight of it?

Write your answers here:

_____

_____

_____

Hint: You're on the wrong track if your answers solely relied on anything outside of your control, such as the addition of more nurses on an understaffed unit, or your coworker not bristling when you tell him you are going on your meal break, or even your cat not waking you at 3 AM because he's bored and wants to play with your hair.

LOOKING AT YOUR RESPONSE TO STRESS

While it would certainly make things easier and a lot less stressful if these situations and others could happen according to your needs, wishes, and desires, as you surely know, this is not always the case. Of course, it is often important to have your voice heard, to assert your needs, to take action. And, there are times when speaking up or taking direct action on your own actually results in what is needed to reduce the strain: a new nurse is oriented, the coworker remembers not to complain when you take your breaks, and the cat… well, two out of three isn't bad!

While it may sound trite (because you may have heard it so many times and perhaps never believed it), the answers to these questions often lie within you, or at the very least, involve you and not always others. It is quite possible, given the right skills, enough motivation, and perhaps a bit of support, to feel less stressed, or perhaps not stressed at all, even if the situation (too few nurses, bristly coworkers, and bored cats) causing your distress remains unchanged.

Change and stress are highly personal experiences. Other people may not experience a situation you find stressful in the same way. Your lifetime of experiences, your personal history, colors the perception you have of events and determines whether or not you will feel distressed by them. The source of stress lies not in the event itself, but rather in your unique perceptions of it, along with the expectations you have, and the meaning this situation has for you.

As you recall from Chapter 1, this pressure can escalate into a crisis, a state in which familiar patterns of thinking, behaving, and responding become ineffective, leading to a state of dysfunction. The word *crisis* is taken from the Greek word *krinein*, which means turning point, a place of departure that leads either to the potential for growth, or to stagnation, or to retreat/regression, depending your ability to recognize the opportunity in this turning point and use it on your behalf.

All stressful events are accompanied by a heightened state of alertness, a hyper-vigilance, an abundance of energy, often experienced as "nervous energy," a state of anxiety, of arousal. Your challenge is to harness this energy and transform it into a productive effort on your behalf so that you can take advantage of the opportunities available in the crisis you are facing. To do this requires a willingness to look inward.

Because your reaction to stress is personal, is within you (as it is with each individual), and because whether or not stress escalates into a crisis is influenced by what you see and do, it follows that it must be understood and handled from that place as well.

This in no way excuses others from the responsibility they have for the situations that are likely to induce stress, for example, the healthcare administrator who refuses to deal with a physician's disruptive behavior or who enforces a policy of mandatory overtime as the only solution to the nursing shortage. Nor does this imply that all there is to do when faced with stressful situations is to "go within" and do nothing "outer" about it.

What this means instead, is that as long as you keep the focus on what you can control, namely yourself, rather than others, you have leverage for managing a previously unmanageable situation, even if it doesn't change, as well as the choice to decide whether you want to do something directly about it yourself, or support the efforts of others to do so.

WHAT MAKES NURSING PRACTICE STRESSFUL?

Working Conditions

When nurses are surveyed about their work, they typically report feeling more stressed by their working conditions than by the patients they care for. In the online version of *The Detroit Free Press* (*freep.com*), Bill Bergstrom in "Almost Half of Nurses Near Burnout, Study Shows" (May 7, 2001) cites growing patient loads, understaffing and verbal abuse as sources of stress in nursing. He quotes a survey published in the May–June 2001 issue of the policy journal *Health Affairs* that must surely be ringing loud alarm bells across the nation:

> "One of every three U.S. nurses surveyed younger than age 30 planned to leave their jobs within the next year, with more than 43 percent scoring high on a burnout inventory used to measure emotional exhaustion and the extent to which they felt overwhelmed by work. More than half said they had been subjected to verbal abuse."[2]

In this same article, Linda Aiken, the director of the University of Pennsylvania School of Nursing's Center for Health Outcomes and Policy Research, used the term "ward rage" to describe the degree of frustrated helplessness many nurses are currently experiencing because of persistent organizational problems heightened by the nursing shortage in which nurses are working longer hours with less help.

When nurses are unable to meet the responsibilities they have to their patients according to standards of nursing practice they were taught, and to which they are held legally accountable, an unsolvable and therefore highly stressful conflict is created for them. Clearly, during this current nursing shortage, talked about as a crisis in the healthcare industry that is anticipated to increase in severity in the years to come, this cause of nursing stress needs to be taken seriously by healthcare administrators, nursing associations, and government agencies in order to preserve the current nursing workforce as well as recruit more nurses. Individual nurses need to, and indeed are, taking this situation seriously as well, as evidenced by what is for many of them the heart-breaking decision to leave nursing rather than participate in the continued compromise of patient care. Refer to Chapter 3, "The State of Nursing Practice," for additional discussions about nursing practice environments, working conditions, and what is being done about them.

Habituated Responses

While the conditions in which the nurse works have become greatly intensified by the present nursing shortage, they have been a persistent source of stress in nursing practice for decades. Often, nurses respond to these working conditions by developing patterns of behavior that tend to compound and amplify their already stressful situation. In an attempt to maintain safe and effective patient care in understaffed hospitals, they work in a heightened state of alertness and vigilance during long shifts of eight to twelve hours, often without taking enough breaks to restore their energy and frequently staying overtime to finish documentation and paperwork. Torn between the needs of their patients and their own needs for adequate nutrition, hydration, and rest, they bypass common sense and make the choice for the other person over themselves.

Consider the situation described below to determine how automatically you might respond to the needs of others even if you know it's not the right action to take:

Imagine that you are on an airplane, traveling with a six-year-old boy, someone who is too young to take care of himself and for whom you are therefore responsible. You've been in the air for about two hours and have settled down to a well-earned rest after a hectic morning of activity. You are awakened from your nap by lights flickering on and off, with the plane being jostled back and forth, as it flies through a thunderstorm. Suddenly the oxygen masks the flight attendants taught you about earlier drop down in front of you. Place a check mark next to the response below that most closely matches what you would do with these masks:

1. ❏ I would put the child's mask on first because he can't do this for himself.
2. ❏ I would put my mask on first because unless I do, I may pass out and then the child and I would be without oxygen.
3. ❏ I know I should put my mask on first but my instinct is to put the child's on first and it's hard to know if I could override this automatic behavior.

The correct answer, of course, is number 2. However, many people find themselves more closely aligned with number 3, knowing what they should do but torn about their ability to do it. If your response was number 1, answering unequivocally and immediately, hardly allowing for the possibility that there could be another answer, your attention to the needs of others at the exclusion of your own needs could benefit from a bit of self-reflection.

Many nurses work without their "oxygen," which is a symbolic representation of their physical, mental, emotional, spiritual, and interpersonal needs They run around making sure everyone, their patients especially, have their masks on, get their needs met, but often neglect their own, even as they realize it's wrong.

Managers and administrators who are squeezed tight by the economic restraint of managed care implicitly or explicitly reinforce these unhealthy behaviors. They refuse or are seemingly helpless to do anything different, although the sounds of "ward rage" from frustrated nurses who have reached their limit, along with the threat of their mass exodus, is beginning to get their attention of late.

As if this weren't enough, there is yet an additional factor that reinforces the behavior of nurses overriding their needs in favor of others. When nurses, who are 95 percent women, do professional work that is, by definition, focused on the needs of others and then continue this other-focused pattern of behavior in their personal lives in the form of caring for children and families, they increase the likelihood of developing habits of behavior that leave their own needs persistently secondary to the needs of others. This alone is a prescription for burnout. Add to this a huge dose of compassion fatigue to which all helping professionals are prone, men and women alike, and you have people in great need of personal and professional resuscitation and life support.

Compassion Fatigue

Nurses are healers who use their skills as relationship-builders in a cycle of caring that requires them to connect and disconnect, attach and detach to others, *many, many* others, in the course of a day, a week, over the years, and in a lifetime of work.

This cycle of caring can be as exhilarating as it is exhausting, and as satisfying as it is stressful. As a result, they (along with others in the helping professions, such as psychologists and social workers) are highly prone to compassion fatigue, a type of burnout that is characterized by a loss of the ability to connect with or care about the emotional experiences of patients, or other people in their life.

A kind of emotional numbness replaces the natural animation that once existed in their response to the needs of others, resulting in the avoidance of these kind of situations or a kind of robotic, going-through-the-motions response that is a compromise solution: Nurses continue in their work but are no longer able to experience or express the compassion they once had. They join the ranks of the "walking wounded," continuing to work, but feeling too stressed or too exhausted to care.

Compassion fatigue happens when nurses become overwhelmed with the intensity of the emotional experiences of others and with what it takes for them to respond in a caring, supportive way. It is not that they don't know how to respond, but rather that they are being asked to respond to too many patients who most likely also require high-tech interventions. However, it is not always the simultaneity of "high-touch" and "high-tech" that is the problem; many nurses at the expert level of practice have seamlessly woven together these two components of care with great mastery, ensuring that the compassion essential to patient care is preserved. Rather, the problem is the volume of patients nurses are asked to care for, especially in understaffed healthcare settings, as well as the insufficient recovery time from these intense experiences.

This dilemma leads to stressful and unresolvable conflicts, or to the often heart-breaking decision to leave nursing altogether. It is poignantly demonstrated in the following poem written by a nurse who chose to remain anonymous. The poem was a response to another well-known poem called *Crabbit Woman*, which you can read at *pennyparker2.com/crabbit.html*.

Nurse's Response to Crabbit Old Woman

What do we see, you ask, what do we see?
Yes, we are thinking when looking at thee!
We may seem to be hard when we hurry and fuss,
But there's many of you, and too few of us.

We would like far more time to sit by you and talk,
To bathe you and feed you and help you to walk,
To hear of your lives and the things you have done;
Your childhood, your husband, your daughter, your son.
But time is against us, there's too much to do
Patients too many, and nurses too few.
We grieve when we see you so sad and alone,
With nobody near you, no friends of your own.
We feel all your pain, and know of your fear
That nobody cares now your end is so near.

But nurses are people with feelings as well,
And when we're together you'll often hear tell
Of the dearest old Gran in the very end bed,
And the lovely old Dad, and the things that he said,
We speak with compassion and love, and feel sad
When we think of your lives and the joy that you've had.

When the time has arrived for you to depart,
You leave us behind with an ache in our heart.
When you sleep the long sleep, no more worry or care,
There are other old people, and we must be there.
So please understand if we hurry and fuss—
There are many of you, and too few of us.

—Anonymous[3]

BURNOUT AND BURNOUT PROTECTION

Burnout is a form of mental, physical, emotional, spiritual, and interpersonal exhaustion that is not easily restored by sleep or rest. It is characterized by an inability to balance the demands placed on you with your capacity to meet them. Burnout results when stress management strategies fail. Nurses experience burnout as the result of feeling overwhelmed and unable to cope with the day-to-day stress of their work over a long period of time, during which they typically move from being enthusiastic caregivers to apathetic "robots," sometimes referred to as the "walking wounded." These are the nurses who are in varying degrees of "going through the motions" of their professional and personal lives, often apathetic or bitter, many wounded from the experience of caring too much about others, without knowing how to care about and for themselves simultaneously. These are most likely the nurses who are having difficulty balancing the nurse-patient-caring equation discussed in Chapter 1.

Valerie J. Nelson, in "Nurses and Burnout" (*nurseweek.com/features/97-2/burn.html*), reports that Mickey Bumbaugh, a senior counseling specialist at M.D. Anderson Hospital in Texas:

> ". . . . thinks it's time to update the aging term (burnout), which was borrowed from the space industry. Instead of focusing on 'avoiding burnout,' she prefers to think of it as 'learning to stay well.' She goes on to say that 'The secret to having enough energy to keep giving compassionate care lies in creating a positive environment *within yourself . . . don't forget to take care of yourself.*'"(italics added)[4]

SUCCEEDING AND THRIVING AS A NURSE IN CHALLENGING TIMES

How, then, are we to succeed as nurses, indeed as people, in these challenging times of change and amid the crisis of a nursing shortage we are warned will be unlike any other? Is it possible to sustain our strength, energy, and motivation while being bombarded with so much information, so many tasks, so many demands, and so much responsibility?

What does it takes to succeed, to meet these challenges, to see the "turning points" in them, and perhaps use them as launch pads for our development and growth? Is this even possible? *It is not only possible, it is essential!* Essential to the individual nurse, essential to the profession as a whole, and essential to the patients the nurse cares for.

When a situation that causes distress cannot be readily changed, or when the solution is too far into the future to seem to matter, what is left to do is relate to the situation differently. What is left to do is to alter the meaning it has for you; to exploit some part of it on your own behalf; to take charge of what you can, namely yourself, and use the situation to your benefit. What is left to do is to take care of yourself through it.

This kind of self-focus and self-reliance translates into a stance called self-care. It is this stance, this commitment to and individual responsibility for preserving and conserving one's mental, emotional, and physical resources that is key to surviving and thriving in challenging times. It is one of the three indispensable legs of the three-legged stool of your nursing success. (See Chapter 1.)

To decline your responsibility for self-care is to ignore the contribution you may be making to being off-balance and incapacitated. To not recognize your need for self-care may be contributing to your burnout and to the extinguishing of your passion for nursing.

EMPOWERMENT AND RESILIENCE

Empowerment and resilience are not necessarily something you learn, but rather a capacity that results from something you do, namely, self-care. It is the commitment you make to yourself to ensure that your energy and resources are preserved, especially during challenging situations.

Empowerment is the refusal to be trapped without options, *no matter what!* Empowerment is *you* in the driver's seat of your life. Rather than following the advertising slogan of the Greyhound Bus Company, "Leave the driving to us,™" the empowered person responds to the call from Volkswagen whose slogan is, "In life there are passengers and drivers. *Drivers wanted!™*"

> **EMPOWERMENT**
>
> The refusal to be trapped without options, NO MATTER WHAT!

Resilience is the capacity to bounce back from a situation that has overstretched or overextended your resources and capacities. It is the restoration of your mental elasticity, physical stamina, emotional buoyancy, spiritual strength, and interpersonal flexibility, all of which represent the holistic totality of your self.

Look at the dictionary definition of the word:

> resilient, **adj.** (*from the Latin, re = back + salire = to jump), 1. bouncing or springing back into shape, position, etc.; elastic. 2. recovering strength, spirits, good humor, etc. quickly; buoyant.*

> **RESILIENCE**
>
> The restoration of your mental elasticity, physical stamina, emotional buoyancy, spiritual strength, and interpersonal flexibility by means of SELF-CARE.

Think of the resilience of a rubber band that when stretched, returns to its original shape and elasticity, able to continue its work of stretching again when needed. Then, think of a rubber band that is overstretched, perhaps for too long, and the loss of resilience that results. Ever have an overstretched rubber band break or snap on you? Does this describe a way you might have felt when overextended or stretched beyond your means?

SELF-CARE AND THE THREE-LEGGED STOOL OF NURSING SUCCESS

Nursing stress and burnout have been written about exhaustively by generations of nurses, administrators, mental health professionals, and stress management experts whose answers and solutions fall into two broad categories. The first category addresses the need to improve the conditions in which the nurse works, by increasing the nurse-patient ratio, for example, or by dealing with physicians' disruptive behavior. The second category (and the focus of this chapter) addresses the environment *within the nurse* who uses skills and strategies that will prevent stress from reaching burnout levels.

Self-care, like stress, is a very personal experience. What feels like self-care to one person may not to someone else. Do you have a personal definition of self-care? Before reading the descriptions below, pause for a moment, consider yours, and write it here:

_____

_____

_____

Self-care includes the capacity for self-awareness and self-management. Self-awareness is the ability to turn inward and hear the murmurs (or shouts) of discontent signaling the need for action on your own behalf. An example might be thirst or the need to decrease your sensory overload after a few hours of intense work. Self-management refers to the skills and strategies you employ to take this action, for example, reprioritizing your schedule or knowing how to respond when your coworker gives you the "evil eye" after you ask him to watch your IVs during your ten-minute break.

Self-awareness and self-management are the building blocks, the foundation of self-care, one of the three skill-sets used by Nurse CEOs of *You, Inc.* to manage the direction and ensure the quality of their self-owned nursing practice. Self-care, along with the other two skill-sets, namely, your professional and clinical skills, and your career management skills form the "three-legged stool of your nursing success."

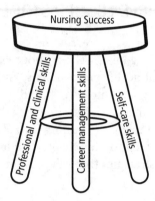

As discussed previously, these three companionate skill-sets are distinct but interrelated and inextricably woven into the fabric of your nursing practice. One without the other leaves your three-legged stool wobbly. All three together, somewhat like the Three Musketeers, create a shield of strength that ensures success.

Some Definitions and Descriptions of Self-Care

Combine the description you wrote with the ones that follow. Allow your understanding of self-care to evolve over time.

Self-care is:

- The capacity to guide and regulate myself, mentally, emotionally, physically, spiritually, and interpersonally, through difficult circumstances utilizing self-awareness and self-management
- An ever-deepening process that engages mind, body, and spirit leading to wholeness
- Stress management I can count on because it involves only me
- Not always expecting something outside of myself to change to feel better
- The conservation of your energy for the preservation of myself
- The antidote to burnout

Obstacles to Self-Care in Nursing

The first obstacle that prevents nurses from making their self-care a priority is their habituated response to the needs of others at their own expense. There seems to be an implicit value system in nursing, often explicitly reinforced by the working conditions common in the healthcare industry, that communicates the idea that it is not possible to achieve a balance between the needs of self and the needs of others. This is not only untrue, it is harmful to the well-being of the nurse and patient alike.

The second obstacle has more to do with the individual nurse, and what it takes to strike a balance between the self and others, irrespective of social and organizational pressures. This involves taking charge of what you can, namely yourself, in order to relate to situations differently. While this might mean mounting an individual protest or supporting the collective efforts of the ANA or your state nurses' association, it also means empowering yourself to ensure that *you* meet your own self-care needs, believing this to be just as essential to the care of your patient as the technical skills that you would never ignore. Since empowerment means the refusal to be trapped without options, NO MATTER WHAT, each nurse must decide what options he or she will exercise on his or her own behalf.

SELF-CARE STRATEGIES FOR BURNOUT PREVENTION

Now that you know (or have been reminded) about how essential it is to take your self-care skills as seriously as your "other-care" skills, the question is, will you?

The self-care strategies that follow are loosely divided into holistic categories that are overlapping, and are certainly not meant to be all-inclusive. Since self-care is always about tuning in to what is most important to you, use this list to whet your appetite for more. Use the print and online resources at the back of this book to obtain more information. Self-care strategies include the following categories:

- Major messages of self-care
- Physical/basic self-care
- Interpersonal self-care
- Mental self-care
- Emotional self-care
- Spiritual self-care

Major Messages of Self-Care

Make Self-Care a Priority

Challenge any beliefs that inhibit your ability to ensure that your needs are met just as you ensure that the needs of others in your life are met.

Recognize That Self-Care Is a Process, Not an Outcome

Self-care is not about perfection but about what you learn and how that changes you in the process of learning it. It is a continual, deepening discovery of who you are and what you need and how best to get it. Your self-care needs change as you grow and develop over time. Your appreciation of your own self-care and your periodic or frequent struggles with it will make you more appreciative of the struggles your patients experience. Model for them the process, the journey of getting there, rather than the potentially intimidating model of perfect self-care.

Know Your Limits

There is a boundary between just enough and too much, perhaps called "good-enough." There is a space that needs to be maintained between demands placed on you and your capacity to meet them. There is a point at which quantity cancels out quality, perhaps a tipping point at which the balance between both disappears and is replaced by a blurred flurry of activity, a mental and physical frenzy that used to be called your life. Is it really true that "you can never have too much of a good thing"? If some chocolate cake is good, can't too much of it make you sick? If some spending gives you pleasure, can't too much spending land you in debt? If some relaxing feels good, can't too much lead to inertia? And, if some work is satisfying, can't too much lead to burnout?

Rise to the Challenge of Change

Expect change. Learn to adapt quickly to what's new and what's next. Learn to live with permanent transition by keeping your well-being self-generated rather than situation-dependent. An example of this is the self-employed attitude of the Nurse CEO of *You, Inc.* who knows that the employer only owns the job he or she has temporarily consented to fill, not the very portable work he or she does.

Perception Is Everything!

It can influence the intensity, duration, and outcome of stressful situations and their potential escalation into crisis states. How you think influences how you feel and eventually how you act. And, it is something over which you have a great deal of control. Remember the pessimist and the optimist, and their respective opinions about the glass being half empty or half filled? It's not so much whether you feel optimistic or pessimistic since both states of mind are natural responses at times. What matters more is that you have the capacity to shift from one state of mind to another, from one way of feeling to another.

Never Abdicate Responsibility for Yourself

Take personal responsibility for maintaining and sustaining your own physical, mental, emotional, spiritual, and interpersonal energy. Expecting others to do so is a prescription for frustration, disappointment, and eventual burnout. Return to the stories of Vicky, Sam, and Nancy from Chapter 1 for a reminder of how to do this (and how not to, as well!).

Treat Yourself with Love and Respect

Be patient and gentle, loving and generous with yourself as you guide yourself through the process of self-care. It's not easy to unlearn patterns of behavior that might be keeping you from doing what you know is in your best interest, for example, learning to say no to additional responsibilities.

Physical Self-Care

Get Your "Oxygen"

Remember the airplane and oxygen mask story earlier in this chapter? Find ways to get *your* symbolic "oxygen" just as you go about your day making sure everyone else gets theirs. This might include nutrition, hydration, rest, and deep breathing as you race down those hallways.

Exercise and Stretch

Include exercising and stretching as a part of your self-care routine. No one needs to remind you of all the health benefits that exercise provides, nor what an essential stress management strategy it is. There is no way to do the rigorous work called nursing without maintaining your physical stamina. Do whatever you have to do to get motivated and then, do it!

Eat Well

Adequate nutrition is essential for your body and mind to function well. It's needed for mental clarity and for protection against fatigue. You know this. You learned it in nursing school. You teach it to your patients. Be sure you listen to yourself as well. Don't fool yourself into thinking you can calculate medication doses or multitask all that technology accurately without it!

Breathe, Breathe, Breathe!

Check in with yourself periodically throughout your busy workday. How are you breathing? Busy people under a lot of pressure (like you!) tend to take shallow breaths, with muscle tension keeping their chest from expanding fully. Put your pathophysiology thinking cap on here: What do you *know* this does to the amount of circulating oxygen required for precise thinking and mental alertness? You would be very concerned if one of your patient's oxygenation was compromised. You would take immediate action. In fact, you would treat this as an urgent situation, perhaps even an emergency. Are you worthy of anything less?

Sleep and Rest

Make sure you sleep enough and rest/nap regularly. Sleep is not a disposable commodity, even though to live and work in today's world, most people act as if it were. Think for a moment: what's often the first thing you do when pressed for time to get a project, (often overdue) done? If your answer is get up earlier or stay up later, you have lots of company, all as sleep-deprived and probably yawning as much as you!

Manage Your Time

Take time management seriously. Recognize that it is just as important to prioritize your schedule as it is to schedule your priorities, and to make sure that you are one of the priorities that gets scheduled into your day. Get a planner or a calendar and use it to ensure that "other-care" needs are attended to and that self-care has a place as well. You are much more likely to get to the gym, shop for nutritious foods, or keep your "play-dates" if they are scheduled into your life.

Interpersonal Self-Care

Detach and Unplug

Detach from others. Slow the pace periodically. Dare to spend a day in your pajamas! Even better, dare to unplug from all the technology you are tethered to and over-stimulated by day in and day out. Imagine that not knowing what is going on in the world for 10 or 12 hours might be more restful than checking on the Nasdaq and Dow Jones Average from your palm pilot or from that ubiquitous "crawl" along the bottom of your TV screen. What do you think this constant alertness and sensory overload does to the catecholamine levels in your blood stream (put your pathophysiology hats on again for this one. Hint, the answer has to do with stress and lower immune functioning).

Seek Solitude

Find a sanctuary for you alone, at home and at work, and use it. Even for five or ten minutes, use it! A space you can go to, however briefly to recenter, ground yourself, and breathe more fully. There are none of these spaces at work, you say? Nonsense! Look around. What about the grounds around the hospital? What about going outside briefly and combining being alone with a little stroll or a fast walk? It's raining, you say? There are bathrooms everywhere. Be creative. This isn't about locking yourself away from your responsibilities for hours on end. This is about taking a few moments and quieting yourself down, treating yourself to a few minutes of solitude to rest and restore so you can do more. If this still sounds impossible, read the next self-care strategy.

Say Yes to Yourself

Learn to say no to others more often in order to say yes to yourself. Establish realistic boundaries that ensure you have your needs met at least as often as you are willing to meet the needs of others, including your patients, your coworkers, and the nurse manager who is desperate and counting on you to stay overtime just one more day this week. If this sounds impossible, take an assertiveness course or consider psychotherapy to figure out why you have such trouble treating yourself with the same consideration and respect you are willing to give to others. For those of you who seem to find it impossible to take your meal breaks, and nothing you've read in this book or elsewhere has so far gotten through to you, consider this additional way to think about it:

> Most organizations do not pay employees for the 60 to 90 minutes that are allotted for meal breaks. For example, if you work from 8 to 4:30 you are most likely getting paid for seven or seven and a half of these hours. When you don't take the allotted time for your breaks, you might as well compute your hourly rate and drop off that amount of money in an administrator's office as a donation to the hospital or healthcare facility you work for. If you do this everyday you work, you are making a substantial donation to this organization and perhaps your tax advisor should be aware! If you are getting overtime pay for working through your meal breaks, you are asked once again to consider the pathophysiological effect this has on your physical and mental well-being.

Don't Play the "Blame Game"

Hold other people responsible for their behavior, not for the feelings you have as a result of that behavior. There is no simple cause and effect to the experience of anger. It doesn't happen as a direct cause of someone doing something that you didn't like. It's much more complicated than that. The source of anger is in the meaning of the situation for the person experiencing it. Blaming someone for how you feel is not just taking the easier way out, it's also an abdication of responsibility for yourself. There's a lot of power in anger when used on your own behalf. Knowing what you want (which is the reason you are angry to begin with) and harnessing the energy of anger to get what you want or give up wanting it, as the case may be, is a lot more empowering. For a wonderful discussion of realigning your understanding of anger in this way, read *The Dance of Anger* by Harriet Lerner, especially the chapter called "Who's Responsible for What, the Trickiest Anger Question of All." (see Resources).

Manage Conflicts, Don't Run from Them

Recognize the value in conflict, which goes a long way to strengthen relationships, not weaken them. Conflict occurs when there are opposing points of view. Hearing how others view things allows you to modify your own view and to grow and learn. Whenever many people are together trying to do something complicated (deliver good patient care, for example), conflict will arise. When it is welcomed in the spirit of hearing opposing views, situations are eventually shaped in a better way than one person's ideas alone could ever do. Explore conflict management strategies that allow you to contribute your ideas as well as hear the ideas of others.

Mental Self-Care

Imitate Willow Trees

If you don't like something, change it. Be proactive. Be assertive. Rally the troops around you. Take charge. Show leadership. And, after all is said and done, if you can't change it, change the way you think about it. Adapt to what is there, not what you wish could be. It's okay to keep working on what it is you want to be different as long as you also accept what is in front of you. This doesn't mean giving up in defeat and accepting a poor situation, but rather making a shorter-term decision to "go with the flow," to imitate flexible willow trees instead of rigid oaks, as you continue your efforts toward the longer-term process of change.

Monitor Your Inner Dialogue

Work towards creating a positive attitude within you. Monitor your self-talk, your inner dialogue, that chattering you hear in your head that accompanies you through your activities. How you think about what you are doing will definitely affect how you feel. For example, as you are trying to learn a complicated procedure, replace "This is so hard; I'll never learn it" with "I know I'll get this if I just stay focused and keep trying. I've learned other complicated procedures. I can learn this one too." Yelling at yourself creates stress and tension and prevents you from learning. You wouldn't yell at patients who were struggling to learn how to give themselves insulin. Neither should you yell at yourself, even if no one but you can hear it.

Use the Power of Affirmations

Consider using affirmations to create a positive and encouraging inner environment. An affirmation is a statement, a series of words, stated in the present tense, that you repeat silently to yourself again and again. The power in an affirmation comes from the repetition of it, which eventually influences what you believe and becomes self-fulfilling. Every nurse has the potential to be great, to excel, to contribute, to have a satisfying and fulfilling career. What contributes greatly to these outcomes is your own belief in it. Try the affirmations below and use the resources at the back of the book to learn more.

"I am proactive and assertive."

"I can prioritize and organize my time well."

"I am able to provide for my self-care needs at work."

Emotional Self-Care

Allow Your Feelings to Strengthen You

Make space for and allow feelings to have a prominent and perhaps private place in your life. You are exposed to and a participant in some of the most powerful human dramas to be found anywhere. It is a myth that nurses get used to the pain and suffering they witness. To get used to it means to detach from it and that only happens when burnout prevents you from being able to be caring and compassionate because it just hurts too much. Pain, yours as well as others, is part of the fullness of life. Feelings unexpressed do not go away. They get transformed into other experiences such as muscle tension, headaches, explosive reactions, overeating, loss of mental clarity, and so on. This is not to suggest that you let your feelings have free rein anytime, anyplace. It is often important to shift from them and focus on the task at hand, something nurses are quite good at. What they are often less good at is shifting back again to those feelings at another time and allowing the release that accompanies the expression of feelings in order to reduce the harmful effect that they can have.

Spiritual Self-Care

Experience the Beauty and Peace of Meditation.

Meditation is so much more than getting quiet and focusing on your breath. It is a restful state in which metabolic rates in the body slow, different from sleep, and actually considered more restful in some ways. Meditation is both a stress management strategy and a personal development tool. There are so many ways to meditate that it would be impossible not to be able to find one to suit you. The beauty of meditation is that when you turn inward and get quiet, you can be with yourself in ways that are impossible as you go through your sensory-overloaded and "other-focused" day. Turning inward allows you to determine how to guide yourself according to what's right for you rather than others. Find someone who meditates and allow them to share how precious an experience meditation is.

Try Prayer

If it fits into your spiritual and religious beliefs, try making prayer a part of your life in a routine way. Many people experience a kind of restful meditative state when praying. Spirituality is about being in the presence of the spirit that is a part of each of us and experiencing its beauty and immense power. Yoga is considered by many to be a spiritual experience, an access way to the spirit through the body. Nursing practice has a spiritual component to it that is separate from the religion of the patient for whom you are caring. You learned this in nursing school. It is true for you too. Try it.

MAKE SPACE FOR YOUR SELF-CARE

This chapter has provided you with a road map to the territory of self-care, which you can explore in more depth at your own pace. Create your own itinerary, staying longer, moving on, returning to explore once again, following where your interests and needs take you. Use the resources in this book and those you may already have around you, find role models and mentors, do whatever it takes to take your self-care skills as seriously as you do your other care skills. Those who journey down this road will go a long way to ensuring that they have the resilience and personal power required for a long and satisfying nursing career.

To remind you to say *yes* to your self, and to make space for your self, consider the following:

The Art of Disappearing

When they say Don't I know you?
say no.

When they invite you to the party
remember what parties are like
before answering.
Someone telling you in a loud voice
they once wrote a poem.
Greasy sausage balls on a paper plate.
then reply.

If they say We should get together
say why?

It's not that you don't love them anymore.
You're trying to remember something
too important to forget.
Trees. The monastery bell at twilight.
Tell them you have a new project.
It will never be finished

When someone recognizes you in a grocery store
nod briefly and become a cabbage.
When someone you haven't seen in ten years
appears at the door,
don't start singing him all your new songs.
You'll never catch up.

Walk around like a leaf.
Know you could tumble any second
Then decide what to do with your time.
(Italics added above)[5]

—Naomi Shihab Nye

PART THREE

Resources

ENDNOTES

Chapter 1: The 21st-Century Nurse

1. "Medicine and Technology: What the Future Means to You: The Next Frontiers." *Newsweek*, 6/24/02.

2. Rhema Ellis, Interview of 2002 Graduates. *The News with Brian Williams*, June 7, 2002.

3. Cataldo, Jackie, "Smoke and Debris." *Journal of the New York State Nurses Association,* Spring/Summer 2002, Volume 33, Number 1.

4. Stevens, Janet, "Someone to Fill My Shoes." *Nursing Spectrum*, June 3, 2002.

5. "The Magnet Nursing Services Recognition Program: Making a Difference—Highlights From 2001." *ANCC Credentialing News*, Spring 2002.

6. "Magnet Hospitals Show the Way." *Report, the Official Newsletter of the New York State Nurses Organization,* June 2002.

7. Naisbitt, John, *Megatrends: Ten New Directions Transforming our Lives.* Warner Books, 1982.

Chapter 2: The World of Nursing Practice

1. Gordon, S., *Life Support: Three Nurses on the Front Lines.* New York: Little, Brown and Company, 1997.

2. Nightingale, F., *Notes on Nursing: What It Is and What It Is Not.* London: Harrison and Sons, London, 1859. (A facsimile edition: Philadelphia: J.B. Lippincott Company, 1946.)

3. Henderson, V., *Basic Principles of Nursing Care*. London: International Council of Nurses, 1961.

4. _____ *Scope and Standards of Advanced Practice Registered Nursing*. Washington, D.C.: ANA, 1996.

5. _____ *Nursing's Social Policy Statement (Second Edition)*. Washington, DC: ANA, 2003.

6. _____ *Standards of Clinical Nursing Practice, Second Edition*. Washington, DC: ANA, 1998.

7. American Nurses Association, *Enhancing Quality of Care Through Understanding Nurses' Responsibilitie*s. Kansas City, MO: ANA,1986.

8. New York State Nurses Association, *Nurses' Rights: Preserving Nursing Practice in Unsafe Client Patient Situations*. Latham: NYSNA, 1997.

9. _____ *Memo for CMA Executive Directors on Nursing's Agenda for the Future*. Washington, DC: ANA, 2002.

10. Buerhaus, P., *News and Views*. Providence: Rhode Island State Nurses Association, Winter 2000.

11. Murray, M., "The Nursing Shortage: Past, Present and Future." *JONA 32*, (2002).

12. Kimball, B. and O'Neil, E., *Health Care's Human Crisis: The American Nursing Shortage*. Princeton, NJ: The Robert Wood Johnson Foundation, 2002.

13. Greenberg, M., "Hailing One of Health Care's Priceless Resources—Nurses." *AMNews*, online, January 28, 2002.

14. _____ *Assessing Your Nursing Practice Environment: A Guide for Nurses Seeking Employment in Health Care Settings*. Latham: NYSNA, Latham, 1997.

15. McClure, M., Poulin, M., Sovie, M., and Wandell, M., *Magnet Hospitals*. Kansas City, MO: American Nurses Association, 1983.

16. _____ *Nursing's Agenda for Health Care Reform*. Washington, DC: ANA, 1993.

Chapter 3: The State of Nursing Education

1. Conner, Daryl R., *Managing at the Speed of Change: How Resilient Managers Succeed and Prosper Where Others Fail.* New York: Random House, 1992.

2. "Faculty Shortages Intensify Nation's Nursing Deficit." American Association of Colleges of Nursing Publications. *aacn.nche.edu/Publications/issues/IB499WB.htm*

3. "A Continuing Challenge: The Shortage of Educationally Prepared Nursing Faculty." American Association of Colleges of Nursing Publications. *nursingworld.org/ojni/topic14/tpc14_3.htm*

4. "Nursing Education's Agenda for the 21st Century." American Association of Colleges of Nursing Publications. *aacn.nche.edu/Publications/positions/nrsgedag.htm*

5. Joel, Lucille, "Education for Entry Into Nursing Practice: Revisited for the 21st Century." *nursingworld.org/ojin/topic18/tpc18_4.htm*

Chapter 5: The Newly Graduated Nurse

1. Benner, Patricia, *From Novice to Expert: Excellence and Power in Clinical Nursing Practice.* New Jersey: Prentice Hall, 2001.

2. Leddy, Susan and J. Mae Pepper, *Conceptual Bases of Professional Nursing.* New York: JB Lippincott Company, 1993.

3. Kramer, Marlene, *Reality Shock.* Massachusetts: Nursing Resources, 1993.

Chapter 6: The Second Career Nurse

1. Trossman, Susan, "Nurses Share Accounts of 9-11 Aftermath." *The American Nurse*, November/December 2001. *nursingworld.org/tan/01novdec/aftermat.htm*

2. Hellinghausen, Mary Ann, "Finding Their Way." *Nurse Week*, December 6, 1999. *nurseweek.com/features/99-12/newprof.html*

3. Engels, Nicholas, "One Solution to the Nursing Shortage." *The Business Journal of Milwaukee*, April 23, 2001. *milwaukee.bizjournals.com/milwaukee/stories/2001/04/23/focus2.html*

4. Quinn, Rose, "Second Sight." *Advance For Nurses*, July 22, 2002. *advancefornurses.com*

Chapter 7: The Older Nurse

1. "Implications of the Older Workforce." House of Delegates Resolution, American Nurses Association Convention, 2002. *nursingworld.org/ pressrel/2002/pr0708.htm*

2. Gabriel, Barbara A., "Wanted: A Few Good Nurses: Addressing the Nation's Nursing Shortage." *AAMC Newsroom Reporter*, Vol. 10, Number 6, March 2001. *aamc.org/newsroom/reporter/march01/nursing.htm*

3. Martinsons, Jane, "Experts Weigh In On Issue of Retaining Older Nurses." *Healthcare Purchasing News Online*, February 2001. *hpnonline.com/inside/ feb01/sb.html*

4. Domrose, Cathryn, "Staying Power." *Nurse Week*, October 22, 2001. *nurseweek.com/extra/sc/reentry.html*

5. Sayewitz, Ronni, "Elder Nurses Tapped to Combat Shortage." *The South Florida Business Journal*, March 4, 2002. *southflorida.bizjournals.com/ southflorida/stories/2002/03/04/story2.html*

6. Frauenheim, Ed, "Grey Matters." *Nurse Week*, January 22, 2001. *nurseweek. com/news/features/01-01/mature.asp*

7. Domrose, Cathryn, "Bridges Across Time." *Nurse Week*, May 14, 2001. *nurseweek.com/news/features/01-05/generations.html*

Chapter 8: Men: The Changing Face of Nursing

1. Wilson, Bruce, R.N., Ph.D., "Men in American Nursing History." *b-wilson. net*

2. "Effective Strategies for Increasing Diversity in Nursing Programs." *American Association of Colleges of Nursing Issues Bulletin*, December 2001. *aacn.nche.edu/Publications/issues/dec01.htm*

3. Williams, Michael, "President's Notes: A Journey of Rediscovery: So How Does It Feel to You?" *AACN News*, August 2001. *aacn.org/AACN/aacnnews. nsf/GetArticle/ArticleThree188?OpenDocument*

4. Williams, Ashleigh and Nikki Battle, "Breakthrough to Nursing." *NYSA Imprint*, Feb./Mar. 2002.

5. Williams, Debra, "Looking For a Few Good Men." *Minority Nurse*, Spring 2002.

6. Evans, Michael, "The Image of Nursing: Past, Present and Future." *NYSA Imprint*, Feb/Mar 2002.

7. "Woodhull Study on Nursing and the Media." Sigma Theta Tau International Honor Society of Nursing. *nursingsociety.org/media/ woodhullextract.html*

8. Snel, Alan, "Paradise Lost No More." *Advance For Nurses*, June 24, 2002

9. Bennet Swingle, Anne, "Still Not Much of a Guy Thing." *Hopkins Nurse* (a publication of the Johns Hopkins Hospital), Fall 2001.

10. "Nurses for a Healthier Tomorrow." Campaign News. *nursesource.org/ campaign_news.html*

11. The Campaign for Nursing's Future." Johnson & Johnson. *discovernursing. com*

12. Rosenstein, Alan H., "Nurse-Physician Relationships: Impact on Nurse Satisfaction and Retention." *American Journal of Nursing*, June 2002.

13. Mason, Diana, "MD-RN: A Tired Old Dance." Editorial, *American Journal of Nursing*, June 2002.

14. Whitman, Walt, "The Wound Dresser." Selections From "Leaves of Grass." New York: Avenel Books (Crown Publishers, Inc.), 1961.

Chapter 9: Becoming the Nurse CEO of *You, Inc.*

1. Bridges, William, *Job Shift: How to Prosper in a Workplace Without Jobs*, New York: Addison-Wesley Publishing, 1994.

2. Saltzman, Amy, "You, Inc." *US News and World Report*, October 28, 1996. *arguscoaching.com/usnews19961028*

3. Noer, David, *Healing the Wounds: Overcoming the Trauma of Layoffs and Revitalizing Downsized Organizations*. San Francisco: Jossey-Bass Publishers, 1993.

Chapter 10: The Product Development Department of *You, Inc.*

1. Hakim, Cliff, *We Are All Self-Employed: The New Social Contract For Working in a Changed World.* San Francisco: Berrett-Koehler Publishers, 1994.

2. Jones, Laurie Beth, *The Path: Creating Your Mission Statement for Work and Life.* New York: Hyperion, 1996.

3. Covey, Stephen R., *The 7 Habits of Highly Effective People.* New York Simon and Schuster, 1990.

4. Perkins-Reed, Marcia, *Thriving in Transition: Effective Living in Times of Change.* New York: Touchstone: Simon and Schuster, 1996.

5. Fritz, Robert, *The Path of Least Resistance.* Fawcett Book Group, 1989.

6. Benner, Patricia, *From Novice to Expert: Excellence and Power in Clinical Nursing Practice.* New Jersey: Prentice Hall, 2001.

Chapter 11: The Marketing Research of *You, Inc.*

1. DeBack, Vivian, "The New Practice Environment" in *Nurse Case Management in the 21st Century*, New York: Mosby, 1996.

2. "Occupational Outlook Handbook." U.S. Department of Labor, Bureau of Labor Statistics, 2002–3 edition. *bls.gov.*

Chapter 12: The Planning Department of *You, Inc.*

1. Benner, Patricia, *From Novice to Expert: Excellence and Power in Clinical Nursing Practice.* New Jersey: Prentice Hall, 2001.

Chapter 14: The Advertising Department of *You, Inc.*: Your Resume

1. Parker, Yana, *The Resume Pro.* Ten Speed Press, 1993.

Chapter 16: The Resilient Nurse: Self-Care Strategies

1. Conner, Daryl R., *Managing at the Speed of Change: How Resilient Managers Succeed and Prosper Where Others Fail.* New York: Random House, 1992.

2. Bergstrom, Bill, "Almost Half of Nurses Near Burnout, Study Shows." *Detroit Free Press*, May 7, 2001. *freep.com/news/health/nurse7_20010507.htm*

3. Author Unknown, "Nurse's Response to Crabbit Old Woman." Penny's Place in Cyberspace. *pennyparker2.com/crabbit.htm*

4. Nelson, Valerie, "Nurses and Burnout: What You Can Do to Prevent It." *Nurse Week. nurseweek.com/features/97-2/burn.html*

5. Shihab Nye, Naomi, "The Art of Disappearing." *Words Under the Words,* 1995.

PRINT RESOURCES

The History of Nursing

Florence Nightingale: Mystic, Visionary, Healer. Barbara Montgomery Dossey, R.N., M.S., H.N.C., F.A.A.N., Springhouse Corporation, 2000. A unique and beautifully illustrated biography of the founder of modern nursing who was a trailblazing social activist, decades ahead of her time.

Nursing, The Finest Art: An Illustrated History. M. Patricia Donahue, Ph.D., R.N., The CV Mosby Company, 1995. A beautifully illustrated history of nursing from ancient to modern times set in its social, political and economic contexts. Documents the alternating presence and absence of men in nursing.

The Changing Healthcare Industry

Nurse Case Management in the 21st Century. Edited by Elaine L. Cohen, Mosby Publishing Company, 1996. An outstanding group of essays packed full of information about the changing healthcare system with contributions from some of the most knowledgeable and influential nurse leaders and futurists, including Tim Porter-O'Grady.

Reengineering Nursing and Healthcare: The Handbook for Organizational Transformation. Suzanne Smith Blancett and Dominick L. Flarey, Aspen Publishers, 1995. This text adapts the framework of the bestselling book, *Reengineering the Corporation* and applies its principles to understanding how and why healthcare is changing from compartmentalized services to more seamlessly integrated systems. Essential for nurse managers and leadership nurses in general, and to all nurses who want an in-depth understanding of the process of hospital and healthcare restructuring.

The Changing World of Work

We Are All Self Employed: The New Social Contract for Working in a Changing World. Cliff Hakim, Berrett-Koehler Publishers, 1994. An excellent guide to shifting from an employee mentality to a self-employed attitude that includes methods of exploring what you want to do, what skills you bring to the marketplace, and who will be most interested in what you have to offer.

To Build the Life You Want, Create the Work You Love: the Spiritual Dimension of Entrepreneuring. Marsha Sinetar, St. Martin's Press, 1995. The sequel to the best-selling and widely read book, *Do What You Love, The Money Will Follow.* This book will help you create work and/or understand the work you do from an inner-development standpoint in which "your consciousness is the doorway to the answers you want."

Managing at the Speed of Change: How Resilient Managers Succeed and Prosper Where Others Fail. Daryl R. Conner, Villard Books, 1994. Provides a structure and a practical approach to change while dealing with the feelings and behaviors common to the change experience. In addition to explaining what is changing and why in the world of work, this book will assist you in understanding the nature and process of change and translate these into specific strategies for coping effectively with stress.

Beat the Odds: Career Buoyancy Tactics for Today's Turbulent Job Market. Martin Yate, Ballantine Books, 1995. A very readable and useful exploration of how to succeed in the changing world of work. Describes what is changing and why and provides practical suggestions for you to use. Topics include why layoffs aren't going to stop and what to do about it, the hot job opportunities, including healthcare, and developing such portable, core career competencies as goal orientation, positive expectancy, inner openness, personal influence, organized action, and informed risk.

C and the Box: A Paradigm Parable. Frank A. Prince, Pfeiffer & Company, 1993. An illustrated story that helps you understand how the conditioning of your past can limit the potential of your future. In an entertaining and creative way, Prince demonstrates the importance of what happens when you get too comfortable with what is familiar.

"The New Deal: What Companies and Employees Owe One Another." Brian O'Reilly, *Fortune*, June 13, 1997. The cover story of this respected business publication explains why loyalty and job security are "nearly dead" and how employers who "deliver honesty and satisfying work can expect a new form of commitment from workers."

Taking Responsibility: Self-Reliance and the Accountable Life. Nathaniel Branden, Simon & Schuster, 1996. An important book for those wishing to broaden and deepen their knowledge of the concept of self-reliance and self-responsibility as it relates to strengthening the self for working and living differently in the 21st century. Written by the psychologist who wrote the classic and best-selling book, *The Psychology of Self-Esteem*.

Job Shift: How to Prosper in a Workplace Without Jobs. William Bridges, Addison-Wesley Publishing Company, 1994. This book is the source of a *Fortune* magazine cover story, "The End of the Job," and describes how organizations are transforming their employment structure from jobs that represent artificial and overlapping divisions of responsibility, to work that needs to be done. Bridges encourages employees to respond to this shift by converting themselves into a business within a market, rather than remain on the payroll of one organization. A clear and concise guide to the facts as well as the psychological impact of "dejobbing," with specific information about how to run the business you have become, which he calls "You & Co."

"You, Inc.", *U.S. News & World Report*, October 28, 1996. A description of how America has "leapt headlong into the information age, and how careers will never be the same." The historical transition about the way in which work is organized and carried out is outlined, along with career profiles of people who have successfully made the transition to self-managing their careers by becoming "You, Inc., the fastest-growing employment segment in the economy."

The Lifetime Career Manager: New Strategies for a New Era. James C. Cabrera and Charles F. Albrecht, Jr, Adams Publishing Company, 1995. A comprehensive review of career planning information with a look at how to manage your career without a guarantee of job security. Challenges the myth of cradle-to-grave employment as it provides tips, guidelines, and ideas for shifting to the new employment reality of self-responsibility.

Liberation Management: Necessary Disorganization for the Nanosecond Nineties. Tom Peters, Alfred A. Knopf, 1992. An outstanding and broad-reaching discussion of how the corporate and business worlds of the 1990s broke themselves into bits and reshaped everything about what they did and how they did it. Topics include why mergers happened, the rise of "contract employment" and how careers started becoming "portfolios of jobs, on and off small and large firms' payrolls."

A Manager's Guide to the Millennium: Today's Strategies for Tomorrow's Success. Ken Matejka and Richard J. Dunsing, American Management Association, 1995. An excellent translation of how organizations will look in the new millennium, and how to learn the new ground rules to "handle, enjoy, and even shape what's in store for you."

Healing the Wounds: Overcoming the Trauma of Layoffs and Revitalizing the Downsized Organizations. David M. Noer, Jossey-Bass Publications, 1993. An indispensable guide to understanding the psychological and interpersonal impact of layoffs on work satisfaction and organizational productivity.

Pritchett and Associates, Inc., 1997. Price Pritchett and his consultancy group publish handbooks based on their training seminars, which cover a wide variety of issues relevant to understanding organizational change and its impact on productivity, interpersonal relationships, and personal stress. Handbook titles include:

- *Firing Up Commitment During Organizational Change*
- *The Stress of Organizational Change*
- *Team Reconstruction: Building a High Performance Work Group During Change*
- *The Employee Handbook for Organizational Change*
- *Culture Shift: Survival of the Fittest, New Work Habits for a Radically Changing World*
- *High Velocity Culture Change: A Handbook for Managers*

Contact: Pritchett and Associates, Inc., 13355 Noel Road, Suite 1650, Dallas, TX 75240; (214) 239-9600; *pritchettnet.com.*

Crisp Publications. Self-study handbooks are published by Crisp Publications for learning about business and personal issues relevant to living and working effectively. Titles include:

- *Managing Personal Change: A Primer for Today's World* by Cynthia D. Scott and Dennis Jaffe

- *Managing Organizational Change: A Practical Guide for Managers* by Cynthia D. Scott and Dennis Jaffe
- *Understanding Organizational Change: Converting Theory to Practice* by Lynn Fossum
- *Managing Disagreement Constructively: Conflict Management in Organizations* by Herbert S. Kindler
- *Personal Time Management* by Marion E. Haynes
- *Managing Anger: Methods for a Happier and Healthier Life* by Rebessa R. Luhn
- *Finding Your Purpose: A Guide to Personal Fulfillment* by Barbara J. Braham
- *Developing Self Esteem: A Guide for Positive Success* by Connie Palladino
- *Developing Positive Assertiveness: Practical Techniques for Personal Success* by Sam R. Lloyd
- *Self-Empowerment: Getting What You Want from Life* by Sam R. Lloyd and Tina Berthelot
- *Empowerment: A Practical Guide For Success* By Cynthia D. Scott, Ph.D., M.P.H., and Dennis T. Jaffe, Ph.D.
- *Effective Networking: Proven Techniques for Career Success* by Venda Rahy-Johnson

Contact: Crisp Publications, Inc., 1200 Hamilton Court, Menlo Park, CA 94025; (800) 442-7477; *courseilt.com*.

Trends, Predictions, and Statistics

Power Shift: Knowledge, Wealth, and Violence at the Edge of the 21ˢᵗ Century. Alvin Toffler, Bantam Books, 1990. Written by a world-famous and widely respected futurist and scholar, this book provides an extensive exploration of the tremendous shifts in power taking place globally and locally. Describes what is changing in our culture, why it's changing, and how to rethink choices in a world based on information and knowledge.

Megatrends: Ten New Directions Transforming Our Lives. John Naisbitt, Warner Books, 1986. This classic book is an excellent resource to help you understand how and why we are moving from an industrial to an information society, from institutional help to self-help, and from hierarchies to networking.

Megatrends for Women. Patricia Aburdene and John Naisbitt, Villard Books, 1992. These international social forecasters describe how "the women of the 1990s are challenging the male-dominated status quo, reintegrating female values and perspectives and recasting the social, political, and economic megatrends of the day."

Megatrends 2000: New Directions for Tomorrow. John Naisbitt and Patricia Aburdede, Warner Books, 2000. Follows up on the informative *Megatrends* and *Megatrends for Women*, illustrating how a remarkable number of their controversial predictions are coming true.

The Popcorn Report: Faith Popcorn on the Future of Your Company, Your World, Your Life. Faith Popcorn, Doubleday, 1992. Called the "Nostradamus of Marketing" by *Fortune* magazine, Popcorn explains what the future will look like and how to profit from it.

Clicking: Sixteen Trends to Future-Fit Your Life, Your Work, and Your Business. Faith Popcorn and Lys Marigold, Harper Collins, 1996. By the futurist and author of the often-quoted Popcorn Report, this book continues the author's ideas and predictions about the business and personal trends that are and will be shaping every aspect of our lives.

Workplace 2000: The Revolution Reshaping American Business. Joseph Boyett and Henry P. Conn, Plume Books, 1991. An excellent description of what the future American workplace will look like and what employees need to do to meet the new demands and expectations. Topics include how middle management will be replaced with self-directed work teams, the difference between managers and leaders, and how and why employees must learn self management.

Occupational Outlook Handbook. United States Department of Labor, Bureau of Labor Statistics, U.S. Government Printing Office, 2001. An essential guide, published annually, to how all occupations have been affected by the dramatic and sweeping changes of the late 1990s, including a listing and description of growth industries such as healthcare.

Career Management: General Information

What Color Is Your Parachute? A Practical Manual for Job-Hunters and Career Changers. Richard Nelson Bolles, Ten Speed Press, 2002. Considered by many to be the classic guide and "bible" of career management across all industries, this book is updated annually with a new edition appearing each November. Use this book to identify and utilize your skills more effectively whether you are job hunting or want to be more marketable in your current place of employment.

Resumes! Resumes! Resumes!, Second edition, Career Press, 1996. Top career experts from a variety of fields discuss and demonstrate how to compose effective resumes. In addition to information about the art of writing and editing a resume, this book provides many samples from which to style your resume.

I Could Do Anything If I Only Knew What It Was: How to Discover What You Really Want and How to Get It. Barbara Sher, Dell Books, 1995. A guide and sourcebook for overcoming the blocks that prevent you from engaging in the work you want to be doing. This book takes you through a process of self-exploration, including action-oriented goal setting.

Writing That Works: How to Write Effective E-Mails, Letters, Resumes, Presentations, Plans, Reports, and Other Business Communications. Kenneth Roman and Joel Raphaelson, Harper Information, 2000. This book contains especially helpful sections on email and e-writing to ensure professionalism and political correctness.

E-Resumes: Everything You Need To Know About Using Electronic Resumes to Tap into Today's Hot Job Market. Susan Britton Whitcomb and Pat Kendall, McGraw Hill, 2001. An A-Z guide for job seeking in the 21st century with special emphasis on how to construct, post, attach and send electronic resumes.

Finding a Path With Heart: How to Go from Burnout to Bliss. Beverly Potter, Ronin Publishers, 1995. A practical sourcebook that describes how to find work satisfaction, packed with entertaining and useful drawings, stories, exercises, and quotes.

Nursing-Specific Career Management

"Creating Your Mission Statement for Work and for Life." Paula Schneider, Nursing Spectrum, Gannett Satellite Information Network, Inc., 1998. Written by a registered nurse who studied with Laurie Beth Jones, author of *The Path: Creating Your Mission Statement for Work and For Life.* This article summarizes the process of creating your mission statement and includes examples of its application to nursing.

What You Need to Know About Today's Workplace: A Survival Guide for Nurses. Lyndia Flanagan, American Nurses Publishing, 1995. In addition to explaining how and why the healthcare industry is changing, this book provides useful information about employment rights and protections (such as collective bargaining, at-will employment, and layoffs), employer terms and conditions of employment (such as performance appraisals, grievance handling, and liability protection), and the management of stress and conflicts in restructuring environments. There is an extensive appendix with sources of information on employment rights and protections as well as a comprehensive reference list and bibliography.

Resumes for Nursing Careers. (no author) McGraw Hill, 2001. Contains sample resumes and cover letters for nurses, including tips and worksheets to simplify the process.

Nursing Spectrum 2001–2002 Career Fitness Guide. Gannett Satellite Information Network, Inc. This excellent resource is published annually by Nursing Spectrum. The many nationwide advertisements provide you with excellent information about the features, professional climate, and changing purpose and structure of the organizations. This periodical will prove very useful as healthcare continues to restructure, and contains important addresses and phone numbers. In addition, there are many useful career-oriented articles.

The Pfizer Guide: Nursing Career Opportunities. Published for the Pfizer Laboratories, Pratt, and Roerig divisions of Pfizer, Inc., by Merritt Communications, 1994. Edited by Mary O. Mundinger. A compendium of over 50 nursing career profiles written by nurses who specialize in each of the roles they write about. Contains detailed information about the role, practice environments, and qualifications necessary to pursue each as a career path.

Reinventing Your Nursing Career: A Handbook for Success in the Age of Managed Care. Michael Newell and Mario Pinardo, Aspen Publications, 1998. Describes how and why nursing and healthcare is changing with special emphasis on managed care opportunities and the healthcare industry as a consumer-driven business environment.

Managing Your Career in Nursing. Frances C. Henderson and Barbara O. McGettigan, National League for Nursing Press, 1994. Provides specific and very detailed descriptions about traditional and emerging nursing practice options and opportunities, including self-assessment tools for practically every topic discussed. Nursing novices as well as seasoned professionals who seek a detailed understanding of nursing roles will find this book helpful.

Career Planning for Nurses. Betty Case, Ph.D., R.N., Delmar Publishers, 1997. An informative guide in career management and self-assessment to assist nurses in creating opportunities for blending their strengths with marketplace needs. Contains a special section for student nurses and an excellent chapter on the nurse informatics role.

Self-Care, Stress Management, Personal Growth

Nursing Specific

Holistic Nursing: A Handbook for Practice, Second Edition. Barbara Montgomery Dossey and Lynn Keegan, Aspen Publications, 1995. This is a stress management book disguised as a nursing textbook. Its approaches are useful not only for coping with stress in general, but with the particular kind of stress inherent in nursing practice. Packed with information about wellness, the psychophysiology of body-mind healing, nutrition, relaxation strategies, imagery, the authors assist you in consulting the truth within, and from that vantage point reach out more effectively to patients.

Healing Yourself: A Nurse's Guide to Self-Care and Renewal. Sherry Kahn and Mileva Saulo, Delmar Publishers, Inc., 1994. A concise and comprehensive handbook with holistic approaches that are practical and easy to use in order to sustain your "body, mind, and spirit as you meet the daily demands of your challenging career."

Pro-Nurse Handbook: Designed for the Nurse Who Wants to Survive/Thrive Professionally. Melodie Chenevert, Mosby, 1993. An entertaining and useful guide to understanding and managing the personal and interpersonal problems that lead to the loss of work satisfaction and sometimes to burnout. Topics include learning to pace yourself, ways to increase your work satisfaction, dealing with procrastination, and understanding the "business" of nursing.

General

The 7 Habits of Highly Effective People: Powerful Lessons in Personal Change. Stephen R. Covey, Simon & Schuster, 1990. A well-known and widely read classic that presents a "principle-centered" approach for solving professional and personal issues.

Principle-Centered Leadership. Stephen R. Covey, Summit Books, 1991. Explores issues of personal development that lead to spending your time around self-identified principles rather than the priorities of others.

First Things First. Stephen R. Covey, A. Roger Merrill, and Rebecca R. Merrill, Simon & Schuster, 1994. A time-management book that expands on and specifies Covey's time-management description in *The 7 Habits of Highly Effective People.* Correlates time management with vision, roles, and empowerment principles.

Developing a 21st Century Mind. Marsha Sinetar, Villard Books, 1991. This best-selling author of *Do What You Love, the Money Will Follow* describes a process she calls positive structuring, the necessary path to shifting from the traditional mind—which Sinetar argues is fear-motivated, dualistic, and egocentric—to the nondualistic and synergistic 21st-century mind needed for living successfully as the world changes.

Emotional Intelligence: Why It Can Matter More Than IQ. Daniel Goleman, Bantam Books, 1995. This book has become a classic in its field, and presents ground-breaking behavioral research that explains and demonstrates how emotional intelligence is essential to self-awareness, impulse control, self-discipline, persistence, self-motivation, and empathy.

The Fifth Discipline Fieldbook: Strategies and Tools for Building a Learning Organization. Peter Senge, Currency and Doubleday Books, 1994. A beautifully conceived and organized book based on Senge's classic work, *The Fifth Discipline.* Topics include reinventing relationships, building vision, developing personal mastery, and systems thinking.

The Path of Least Resistance: Learning to Become the Creative Force in Your Own Life. Robert Fritz, Fawcett Columbine Publishers, 1989. Explains how to move into your future vision by understanding your present reality and using the creative tension between these two experiences to create the momentum you need to get where you want to go.

Women Who Run With the Wolves: Myths and Stories of the Wild Woman Archetype. Clarissa Pinkola Estes, Ballantine Books, 1992. This book invites you to experience the powerful force within you that is "natural, creative, powerful, filled with good instincts, and ageless knowing." Nurses will especially identify with the chapter called "Homing: Returning to OneSelf."

Revolution from Within: A Book of Self-Esteem. Gloria Steinem, Little, Brown, and Co., 1992. An autobiographical account of this feminist's life and journey, primarily from the standpoint of her own personal development, describing the necessary "revolution of spirit and consciousness," which she had always assumed was secondary to social change.

A Passion for the Possible: A Guide to Realizing Your True Potential. Jean Houston, Harper San Francisco, 1997. Creates an understanding of how to break free from the limiting beliefs that will prevent you from taking advantage of the opportunities change always brings.

Self Renewal: High Performance in a High Stress World. Dennis T. Jaffe and Cynthia D. Scott, Crisp Publications, 1994. An extremely useful workbook that contains clear explanations as well as self-assessment tools and self-reflection exercises. Uses a self-care approach to stress management, presenting ways to increase your self-awareness, self-management, and self-renewal strategies.

The Path: Creating Your Mission Statement for Work and for Life. Laurie Beth Jones, Hyperion, 1996. Provides inspiring and practical advice to lead readers through the steps of defining and fulfilling a mission in life. The lessons on creating a mission statement are easily transferable to the world of work.

The Artist's Way: A Spiritual Path to Higher Creativity. Julia Cameron, G. P. Putnam Sons, 1992. An empowering book to increase the creative expression of any and all areas of your life. Engages you in a 12-week personal development journey to "recover your creativity from a variety of blocks, including limiting beliefs, fear, self sabotage, jealousy, guilt, addictions, and other inhibiting forces."

Life Skills: Taking Charge of Your Personal and Professional Growth. Richard J. Leider, Pfeiffer & Company, 1994. Takes a personal development viewpoint to career strategies and work success. Life and work planning are explored in an interactive workbook to "help you align your career objectives, talents, and deepest values."

Use Your Anger: A Woman's Guide to Empowerment. Sandra Thomas and Cheryl Jefferson, Pocket Books, Simon and Schuster, 1996. Written by a nurse and based on a seven-year, nationwide study she conducted, this book will help you understand the impact anger may be having on your life and provides you with ways to transform the energy of anger into productive and empowering action.

Changing for Good: The Revolutionary Program That Explains the Six Stages of Change and Teaches You How to Free Yourself from Bad Habits. James Prochaska, John Norcross, Carlo DiClemente, William Morrow and Co., 1994. A well-organized approach to change with some refreshing reinterpretations that demystify the process and provide clear strategies for effective coping.

Minding the Body, Mending the Mind. Joan Borysenko, Bantam Books, Addison-Wesley Publishers, 1988. Written by a psychotherapist and scientist who is described as a pioneer in the new field of psychoneuroimmunology and the founder of the Mind Body Clinic at the New England Deaconess Hospital, this book provides sound and useful information on managing stress as it explains the important relationship between mind and body.

Resilience: How to Bounce Back When the Going Gets Tough. Frederic Flach, Hatherleigh Press, 1997. A simple stress management guide with easy-to-understand descriptions of how stress happens and how to handle it. Topics include the response to stress at different points in the life cycle, what the resilient personality looks like, and how self-worth is related to resilience.

Kicking Your Stress Habits: A Do-It-Yourself Guide for Coping with Stress. Donald A. Tubesing, Whole Person Associates, 1991. A simple and eminently useful self-study guide to stress and change management, with chapters devoted to perception, beliefs, grief, relationship skills, coping habits, and other topics.

Seeking Your Healthy Balance: A Do-It-Yourself Guide to Whole Person Well-Being. Donald A. Tubesing, Whole Person Associates, 1991. Presents a holistic approach to taking care of yourself in the face of demands and responsibilities of work and family.

Thriving in Transition: Effective Living in Times of Change. Marcia Perkins-Reed, Touchstone Books, Simon & Schuster, 1996. An easy-to-read and extremely useful book that takes a holistic approach to adapting to change, using information from the fields of psychology, organizational development, physics, and spirituality.

Margin: Restoring Emotional, Physical, Financial, and Time Reserves to Overloaded Lives. Richard A. Swenson, NavPress, 1992. This book can help you develop strategies for having too much to do and too little time to do it.

Take Time for Your Life. Cheryl Richardson, Broadway Books, 1999. Strategies for making conscious decisions that affect your life with a section on "extreme self care."

INTERNET RESOURCES

1. Internet Gateways and Portals

Because Web addresses tend to change, and listings on the Internet are frequently added or deleted, it is necessary to verify and update these listings periodically. The Internet gateways or portals listed below will give you annotated, searchable databases for each category in this resource, including direct hyperlinks to your sites of interest. These master lists will also contain additional resources not mentioned in this resource:

- American Nurses Association *nursingworld.org*
- Brownson's Nursing Notes *dianebrownson.tripod.com*
- CyberNurse *cybernurse.com/careers.html*
- Google *directory.google.com/Top/Health/Nursing/Internet/Gateway*

    This is a master list of master lists! An excellent resource that contains 53 other national and international nursing master lists, including the ones listed below, each with their Web address as well as a hyperlink directly to it.

- Medi-Smart Resource Directory *medi-smart.com/nursing.htm*
- Nursing Center *nursingcenter.com/home/index.asp*
- Ultimate Nurse *ultimatenurse.com*
- Welch Web Subject Guides *welch.jhu.edu/internet/nursing.html*

    This is the Johns Hopkins University site for nurses and has a library gateway that includes MEDLINE and CINAHL, in addition to many other useful sites.

2. Professional Associations and Organizations

- American Nurses Association (ANA) *nursingworld.org*

  Constituent Members of the American Nurses Association (alphabetically by state):
  Alabama State Nurses Association *alabamanurses.org*
  Alaska Nurses Association *aknurse.org*
  Arizona Nurses Association *aznurse.org*
  Arkansas Nurses Association *arna.org*
  ANA/California *anacalifornia.org*
  Colorado Nurses Association *nurses-co.org*
  Connecticut Nurses Association *ctnurses.org/*
  Delaware Nurses Association *denurses.org*
  District of Columbia Nurses Association, Inc. *www.dcna.org*
  Federal Nurses Association (FedNA) *nursingworld.org/FedNA*
  Florida Nurses Association *floridanurse.org*
  Georgia Nurses Association *georgianurses.org/*
  Guam Nurses Association: Email: guamnurse@ite.net
  Hawaii Nurses Association *hawaiinurses.org*
  Idaho Nurses Association *nursingworld.org/snas/id*
  Illinois Nurses Association *illinoisnurses.com*
  Indiana State Nurses Association *indiananurses.org*
  Iowa Nurses Association *iowanurses.org*
  Kansas State Nurses Association *nursingworld.org/snas/ks*
  Kentucky Nurses Association *kentucky-nurses.org*
  Louisiana State Nurses Association *lsna.org*
  ANA/Maine *anamaine.org*
  Maryland Nurses Association *marylandrn.org*
  Massachusetts Association of Registered Nurses *marnonline.org*
  Michigan Nurses Association *minurses.org*
  Minnesota Nurses Association *mnnurses.org*
  Mississippi Nurses Association *msnurses.org*
  Missouri Nurses Association *missourinurses.org*
  Montana Nurses Association *mtnurses.org*
  Nebraska Nurses Association *nursingworld.org/snas/cmas/ne*
  Nevada Nurses Association *nvnurses.org*
  New Hampshire Nurses Association *www.nhnurses.org*
  New Jersey State Nurses Association *njsna.org*

New Mexico Nurses Association *www.nmna.org*
New York State Nurses Association *nysna.org*
North Carolina Nurses Association *ncnurses.org*
North Dakota Nurses Association *ndna.org*
Ohio Nurses Association *ohnurses.org/*
Oklahoma Nurses Association *oknurses.com*
Oregon Nurses Association *oregonrn.org*
Pennsylvania State Nurses Association *psna.org*
Rhode Island State Nurses Association *risnarn.org*
South Carolina Nurses Association *scnurses.org*
South Dakota Nurses Association *nursingworld.org/snas/sd/*
Tennessee Nurses Association *tnaonline.org*
Texas Nurses Association *texasnurses.org*
Utah Nurses Association *utahnurses.org*
Vermont State Nurses Association *www.vsna-inc.org*
Virgin Islands State Nurses Association Email: vcgvina@viaccess.net
Virginia Nurses Association *www.virginianurses.com/vna*
Washington State Nurses Association *wsna.org*
West Virginia Nurses Association *wvnurses.org*
Wisconsin Nurses Association *wisconsinnurses.org*
Wyoming Nurses Association *wyonurse.org*

- National Council of State Boards of Nursing, Inc. *ncsbn.org*

  State Boards of Nursing
  (alphabetically by state):
  Alabama Board of Nursing *abn.state.al.us/*
  Alaska Board of Nursing *dced.state.ak.us/occ/pnur.htm*
  Arizona State Board of Nursing *www.azbn.org*
  Arkansas State Board of Nursing *www.arsbn.org*
  California Board of Registered Nursing *rn.ca.gov/*
  Colorado Board of Nursing *www.dora.state.co.us/nursing/*
  Connecticut Board of Examiners for Nursing *www.dph.state.ct.us*
  Delaware Board of Nursing *professionallicensing.state.de.us/*
     boards/nursing/index.shtml
  District of Columbia Board of Nursing (Department of Health)
     dchealth.dc.gov
  Florida Board of Nursing *doh.state.fl.us/mqa/*
  Georgia Board of Nursing *sos.state.ga.us/plb/rn*

Guam Board of Nurse Examiners *nurse.org/gu-index.shtml*
Hawaii Board of Nursing *hawaii.gov/dcca/areas/pvl/boards/nursing*
Idaho Board of Nursing *www.state.id.us/ibn*
Illinois Department of Financial and Professional Regulation *idfpr.com*
Indiana State Board of Nursing Health Professions Bureau *www.in.gov/pla*
Iowa Board of Nursing *state.ia.us/government/nursing/*
Kansas State Board of Nursing *ksbn.org*
Kentucky Board of Nursing *kbn.ky.gov*
Louisiana State Board of Nursing *www.lsbn.state.la.us/*
Maine State Board of Nursing *www.state.me.us/boardofnursing*
Maryland Board of Nursing *mbon.org*
Massachusetts Board of Registration in Nursing *www.state.ma.us/reg/ boards/rn/*
Michigan CIS/Bureau of Health Services *www.michigan.gov/cis*
Minnesota Board of Nursing *nursingboard.state.mn.us/*
Mississippi Board of Nursing *msbn.state.ms.us/*
Missouri State Board of Nursing *pr.mo.gov*
Montana State Board of Nursing *mt.gov/dli/license/bsd-boards/nur_board/ board_page.asp*
Nebraska Health and Human Services System, Department of Regulation and Licensure, Nursing Section *www.hhs.state.ne.us/crl/nursing/ nursingindex.htm*
Nevada State Board of Nursing *nursingboard.state.nv.us*
New Hampshire Board of Nursing *state.nh.us/nursing/*
New Jersey Board of Nursing *www.state.nj.us/lps/ca/medical.htm*
New Mexico Board of Nursing *state.nm.us/clients/nursing*
New York State Board of Nursing *www.op.nysed.gov/nurse.htm*
North Carolina Board of Nursing *ncbon.com/*
North Dakota Board of Nursing *ndbon.org/*
Ohio Board of Nursing *www.nursing.ohio.gov*
Oklahoma Board of Nursing *youroklahoma.com/nursing*
Oregon State Board of Nursing *www.osbn.state.or.us/*
Pennsylvania State Board of Nursing *www.dos.state.pa.us/bpoa/cwp/ view.asp?a=1104&q=432883*
Commonwealth of Puerto Rico Board of Nurse Examiners (787)725-7506
Rhode Island Board of Nurse Registration and Nursing Education *www.health.ri.gov/hsr/professions/nurses.php*
South Carolina State Board of Nursing *www.llr.state.sc.us/pol/nursing*

South Dakota Board of Nursing *www.state.sd.us/don/nursing/*
Tennessee State Board of Nursing *state.tn.us/health*
Texas Board of Nurse Examiners *www.bne.state.tx.us/*
Utah State Board of Nursing *www.commerce.state.ut.us/*
Vermont State Board of Nursing *vtprofessionals.org/opr1/nurses/*
Virginia Board of Nurse Licensure *www.dhp.state.va.us/nursing*
Washington State Nursing Care QualityAssurance
    Commission/Department of Health *fortress.wa.gov/doh/hpqa1/hps6/*
    Nursing/default.htm
West Virginia Board of Examiners for Registered Professional Nurses
    www.wvrnboard.com
Wisconsin Department of Regulation and Licensing *www.drl.state.wi.us/*
Wyoming State Board of Nursing *nursing.state.wy.us/*

Other Professional Nursing Associations

- American Academy of Nursing *aannet.org*
- American Association for the History of Nursing *aahn.org*
- American Association of Colleges of Nursing *aacn.nche.edu*
- American Nurses Credentialing Center *nursingworld.org/ancc/*
- American Nurses Foundation *ana.org/anf/*
- American Organization of Nurse Executives *aone.org*
- Florence Project, Inc. *firrp.org*
- International Council of Nurses *icn.ch/*
- National League for Nursing *www.nln.org*
- National Organization for Associate Degree Nursing *noadn.org*
- Nurses for a Healthier Tomorrow *nursesource.org*
- Sigma Theta Tau International Honor Society for Nurses
    nursingsociety.org

3. Specialty Nursing Organizations and Associations

- Alliance for Psychosocial Nursing *psychnurse.org*
- American Academy of Ambulatory Nurses *aaacn.inurse.com*
- American Academy of Nurse Practitioners *aanp.org*
- American Assembly of Men in Nursing *aamn.org*
- American Assisted Living Nurses Association *alnursing.org*
- American Association of Critical Care Nurses *aacn.org*
- American Association of Neuroscience Nurses *aann.org*
- American Association of Nurse Anesthetists *aana.com*
- American Association of Occupational Health Nurses *aaohn.org*
- American Association of Spinal Cord Nurses *aascin.org*
- American College of Nurse Midwives *acnm.org*
- American College of Nurse Practitioners *ancpweb.org*
- American Holistic Nurses Association *ahna.org*
- American Nephrology Nurses Association *anna.inurse.com*
- American Nursing Informatics Association *ania.org*
- American Pediatric Surgical Nurses Association *www.apsna.org/mc/page.do*
- American Psychiatric Nurses Association *apna.org*
- American Radiological Nurses Association *arna.net*
- American Society For Pain Management Nurses *aspmn.org*
- American Society of Peri-Anesthesia Nurses *aspan.org*
- American Society of Plastic Surgery Nurses *aspsn.org*
- Association of Camp Nurses *campnurse.org*
- Association of Community Health Nursing Educators *achne.org*
- Association of Nurses in AIDS Care *anacnet.org*
- Association of Operating Room Nurses *aorn.org*
- Association of Pediatric Oncology Nurses *apon.org*
- Association of Women's Health, Obstetric & Neonatal Nurses *awhonn.org*
- Dermatology Nurses Association *dna.inurse.com*
- Developmental Disabilities Nurses Association *ddna.bluestep.net*
- Emergency Nurses Association *ena.org*

- Endocrine Nurses Society *endo-nurses.org*
- Hospice and Palliative Nurses Association *hpna.org*
- Infusion Nurses Society *ins1.org*
- International Association of Forensic Nurses *www.forensicnurse.org*
- International Organization of Multiple Sclerosis Nurses *www.iomsn.org*
- International Society of Nurses in Cancer Care *isncc.org*
- International Society of Nurses in Genetics *isong.org*
- Minority Nurses Association *minoritynurse.com*
- National Association of Clinical Nurse Specialists *nacns.org*
- National Association of Hispanic Nurses *thehispanicnurses.org*
- National Association of Independent Nurses *independentrn.com*
- National Association of Neonatal Nurses *nann.org*
- National Association of Nurse Practitioners in Women's Health *npwh.org*
- National Association of Orthopedic Nurses *orthonurse.org*
- National Association of Pediatric Nurse Associates and Practitioners *napnap.org*
- National Association of School Nurses, Inc. *www.nasn.org*
- National Black Nurses Association *nbna.org*
- National Gerontological Nursing Association *ngna.org*
- National Nurses in Business Association *nnba.net*
- National Nursing Staff Development Organization *nnsdo.org*
- New York University John A. Hartford Foundation Institute for Geriatric Nursing *hartfordign.org*
- Oncology Nursing Society *ons.org*
- Renalnet: Nephrology Nurses *renalnet.org*
- Rural Nurses Organization *www.rno.org*
- Society For Vascular Nurses *svnnet.org*
- Society of Gastroenterology Nurses Association *sgna.org*
- Society of Otorhinolaryngology, Head/Neck Nurses *sohnnurse.com*
- Wound, Ostomy and Continence Nurses Society *wocn.org*

4. Professional Certification Resources

- American Nurse's Credentialing Center *nursingworld.org/ancc/*

  Provides board certification at the generalist and advanced practice levels in a variety of clinical and administrative nursing specialties, including informatics.

- Nursing Center *nursingcenter.com/prodev/ce_certification.asp*

  Provides detailed certification information (including hyperlinks) in many clinical and administrative areas of nursing practice.

Certification is also available through the following professional associations:

- American College of Nurse Midwives Certification Council *accmidwife.org*
- Board of Nephrology Examiners, Nursing & Technology *bonent.org*
- Certification Board of Infection Control and Epidemiology, Inc. *cbic.org*
- Certification Board of Perioperative Nursing *cc-institute.org/cert.aspx*
- Medical-Legal Consulting Institute Certification for Legal Nurse Consultants *legalnurse.com*
- National Certification Board for Diabetes Educators *ncbde.org*
- National Certification Corporation (certifies obstetric, gynecologic, and neonatal nurses) *nccnet.org*
- Oncology Nursing Certification Corporation *oncc.org*

5. Clinical Nursing Resources

Note: See student nurse websites in the nursing education section of this resource for many additional clinical resource websites.

Gateways and Internet Portals

Use these gateways to select the clinical resources most useful to you. A sampling of what they have to offer appears below:

- The National Library of Medicine Gateway *gateway.nlm.nih.gov/gw/Cmd*
- Nursing Spectrum Websearch: Anatomy/Pathophysiology
  www.nursingwebsearch.com/category.cfm?cat=ANATOMY
- Thomson Delmar Learning Drug Data Base
  delmarlearning.com/resources/virtual-library.aspx

Additional Websites

- Auscultation Assistant (hear actual heart and breath sounds)
  www.wilkes.med.ucla.edu/intro.html
- Lippincott's Nursing Center *nursingcenter.com/home/index.asp*
- Medline plus *medlineplus.gov*
- Nurses PDR Resource List *nursespdr.com*
- Nursing Care Plans *nursingcareplans.com*
- Online Journal of Issues in Nursing *nursingworld.org/ojin*
- PDA cortex *pdacortex.com/listserv.htm*

  Listservs, newsgroups, and electronic newsletters, including listserv communities (with a nursing-specific link) for those using PDAs (personal digital assistants).

6. Nursing Journals and Publications

Use this gateway to find lists of and hyperlinks to more than 200 national and international nursing journals: *medbioworld.com/med/journals/nurse.html*. The gateways listed in at the beginning of this resource will give you long lists of journals as well.

You can also contact the nursing specialty association of interest to you and subscribe to their specific journal or newsletter (see section 3 of this resource). Many of these publications are online. A sampling of some popular nursing journals follows.

- *The American Journal of Nursing (AJN) (nursingworld.org/AJN)*

  The official journal of the American Nurses Association and therefore an indispensable source of nursing practice information. In addition to news about nursing practice issues, AJN provides comprehensive and in-depth clinical articles, including the ability to earn continuing education units by answering and submitting test questions following some of its articles.

- *Nursing 2006 (nursingcenter.com/)*

  This bimonthly newsletter, published by the American Nurses Association, is an important source of nursing practice news, including political/legislative issues, employment practices, workplace issues, and convention news.

- *Report (nysna.org)*

  This official newsletter of the New York State Nurses Association contains state-wide information about nursing practice issues. Each state nurses association publishes an official newsletter with a different title.

- *Calendar (nysna.org/districts/13.htm)*

  This official newsletter of the New York Counties Registered Nurses Association, District 13 of the New York State Nurses Association contains district-wide information about nursing practice issues. Each state nurses association is divided into a number of districts and each publishes an official newsletter with a different title.

- *Nursing Spectrum (nursingspectrum.com)*

  This is the New York metropolitan area's version of an employment and career-oriented publication that is circulated under different names in other areas of the country. This publication is available free to all licensed professional nurses. It contains employment opportunities and career/ workplace information that will help you keep abreast of changes and issues in nursing practice and healthcare.

- *Nurse Week (nurseweek.com/newsletter)*

  Employment opportunities and career information published biweekly for the California area.

- *Advance For Nurses (nursing.advanceweb.com/main.aspx)*

  Available free to all registered nurses, the focus of this biweekly publication includes employment opportunities and articles of general interest to nurses, including professional practice and clinical issues.

- *ICUs and Nursing Web Journal (nursing.gr/index1.html)*

  A peer-reviewed electronic journal

- *American Association of Occupational Health Nurses Journal (aaohn.org/ practice/journal/index.cfm)*

- *Online Journal of Issues in Nursing (nursingworld.org/ojin/)*

- *Online Journal of Nursing Informatics (eaa-knowledge.com/ojni/#)*

- *RN Magazine (rnweb.com)*

- *Nursing Management (nursingcenter.com/)*

7. Nursing Education Resources

Schools and Colleges of Nursing

For information about becoming a registered professional nurse, access the following gateway-type website: *nursing.about.com/cs/aboutnursing/index.htm*.

- American Association of Colleges of Nursing *(AACN) www.aacn.nche.edu*
  Provides comprehensive information on all aspects of nursing education, including lists of and links to colleges and schools of nursing.
- Accelerated B.S.N. or generic Master's programs *www.aacn.nche.edu/Publications/issues/Aug02.htm*

Online/Distance Learning Programs

- "Distance Education: A Consumer's Guide," Western Cooperative For Educational Telecommunications. *wcet.info/resources/publications/conguide/*
- Drexel University e-Learning *drexel.com*
- Duquesne University *nursing.duq.edu/gradOnl.html*
- Jacksonville University School of Nursing *jacksonvilleu.com*
- The State University of New York at Stony Brook *sunysb.edu/spd/online/index.html*
- The University of Phoenix *uopxonline.com*

Student Nurse Support

- American Association of Colleges of Nursing *www.aacn.nche.edu*
- APA style for writing, publication of papers *apastyle.org*

Information on accredited nursing school programs, financial assistance, etc.:

- National League for Nursing *www.nln.org*
- National Student Nurse Association *www.nsna.org*
- Student Nurse Forum *kcsun3.tripod.com*
- Student Nurses.com *studentnurses.com*
- For finding a mentor contact the "Nurses Nurturing Nurses" (N3 for short) at the Academy of Medical-Surgical Nurses *www.medsurgnurse.org/cgi-bin/WebObjects/AMSNMain.woa*

Second Career Nurses

For insightful profiles and information about nursing as a second career:

- "Finding Their Way." Mary Ann Hellinghausen, *NurseWeek*, December 6, 1999, *nurseweek.com/features/99-12/newprof.htm*
- "One Solution to the Nursing Shortage: Second Career Trainees." Nicholas Engels, *The Business Journal of Milwaukee. milwaukee.bizjournals.com*
- "Second Sight." Rose Quinn, *Advance for Nurses*, 7/22/02 *nursing.advanceweb.com/main.aspx*

NCLEX-RN® Exam Resources

National Council of State Boards of Nursing provides important application and qualification information, including a list of its 50 affiliating State Boards of Nursing; see *ncsbn.org*

Test preparation assistance and information

- Kaplan Test Prep—NCLEX-RN® exam *kaplannursing.com*

Continuing Education

Two distance learning options for continuing education are nursing journals and online nursing websites. See the list of nursing journals and publications in section 6 of this resource. This partial list of Internet gateway sites will lead you to an infinite number of continuing education opportunities:

- *Advance for Nurses nursing.advanceweb.com/main.aspx*
- American Nurses Association *nursingworld.org*
- Hospital Soup *hospitalsoup.com*
- Nursing Center *nursingcenter.com/home/index.asp*
- Nursing Spectrum *nursingspectrum.com*
- RnCeus.com *rnceus.com*
- State Nurses Associations (see section 2 of this resource)
- SUNY Stony Brook School of Nursing *www.nursing.stonybrook.edu*
- Ultimate Nurse *ultimatenurse.com*

Financial Assistance

- Nursing Spectrum is one of many Internet gateways that have financial aid and scholarship information: *www.nursingwebsearch.com/*

8. Healthcare Associations and Government Organizations

Use one of the Internet gateways or portals listed at the beginning of this resource to find comprehensive lists of government and healthcare organizations and associations. Some are included below:

- American Academy of Pediatrics *aap.org*
- American Hospital Association *aha.org*
- American Psychological Association *apa.org*
- American Public Health Association *apha.org*
- Centers for Disease Control and Prevention (CDC) *www.cdc.gov*
- Health Insurance Portability and Accountability Act *cms.hhs.gov/ hipaagainfo/01_overview.asp*
- Joint Commission on Accreditation of Healthcare Organizations *jointcommission.org*
- Mayo Clinic *mayoclinic.com*
- Office of Advancement of Telehealth *telehealth.hrsa.gov*
- The American Diabetic Association *diabetes.org*
- The American Heart Association *americanheart.org*
- The American Medical Association *ama-assn.org*
- The American Psychiatric Association *psych.org*
- The American Red Cross *redcross.org*
- The Food and Drug Administration *www.fda.gov*
- The National Institute of Health *www.nih.gov*
- The World Health Organization *who.int/en/*
- To check the status of pending or passed legislation *nursingworld.org/gova/state.htm*
- U.S. Department of Labor Bureau of Labor Statistics *Occupational Outlook Handbook* (published annually) *stats.bls.gov/oco*
- U.S. Department of Health and Human Services Office of Disease Prevention and Health Promotion *healthfinder.gov*

9. Nursing Community and Networking Sources

Listservs, Newsgroups, and Chat Rooms

Master lists and links can be found at many sites including *nursingworld.org.*

General Nursing Listservs
- *nurseweek.com*
- *nursingspectrum.com/nursecommunity/index.htm*

Specialized Listservs
- Breast Cancer *majordomo@redbank.net*
- Case Managers *Casemgr@cue.com*
- Heart Talk *listserv@maelstrom.stjohns.edu*
- Nursing informatics *listserv@lists.umass.edu*

Nursing Chat Rooms
- *virtualnurse.com/chat/index.php*
- *allnurses.com/forums/chatlogin.php*

Nursing Websites

These and many others like them (see section 1 of this resource) offer a kind of "one-stop shopping" experience. They are often gateway-type sites, opening the Internet doors to cyberspace travel to intended destinations and unanticipated surprises.
- All Nurses *allnurses.com*
- Brownson's Nursing Notes *members.tripod.com/~DianneBrownson/*
- CyberNurse *cybernurse.com/careers.html*
- HospitalSoup.com *HospitalSoup.com*
- Nursing Center *nursingcenter.com/home/index.asp*
- *Nursing Spectrum nursingspectrum.com*
- The Student Nurse Forum *kcsun3.tripod.com*
- Ultimate Nurse *ultimatenurse.com*

10. Career Management

Employment

- Monster.com *monster.com*
- *Nursing Spectrum nursingspectrum.com*
- *The New York Times jobmarket.nytimes.com/pages/jobs*

Resumes and Cover Letters

- Career Journal *jobstar.org*
- Kaplan Career Center *kaptest.com*
- Monster.com *resume.monster.com/writingservices/index.asp?msource=HP_v1*

Interview Assistance

- Monster.com *interview.monster.com/virtualinterview*

Job Fairs

- *jobsearch.about.com/library/blfairtip.htm*

11. Self-Care and Stress Management Resources

Use any of the Internet gateways or portals listed in section 1 of this resource to find voluminous listings on stress management and self-care. These additional Internet gateways are specific to stress management and contain long lists of hyperlinks:

- Caring for the Nurse *care-nurse.com*

  Described as "a nursing hideaway, planned just for you," this site offers networking via a listserv and tips for managing stress.

- Holistic-Online.com *holistic-online.com/stress/stress_home.htm*
- Rx for Sanity *rxforsanity.com*
- Stress and Burnout *medi-smart.com/stress.htm*
- Virtual Stress Library *dialogical.net/stress/index.html*

12. Computer and Internet Resources

- *Nurses Guide to the Internet, Third Edition.* Leslie H. Nicholl, Lippincott, 2000.
- *Internet Resources for Nurses.* Joyce Fitzpatrick and Kristen Montgomery, Springer Publishing Co., 2000.
- "Nursing and the Internet," an undergraduate nursing course taught by Margo Thompson, Ed.D., R.N. *webster.edu/~thompsma/internet/index.html*
- Nursing Informatics *www.library.umc.edu/TopicTracks/tt-nursinform.html*
- *Nursing Informatics.* Barbara Carty, Springer Publishing Co., 2000.
- *The Official Smiley Dictionary, smileydictionary.com*
- Webopedia, an online dictionary of computer and Internet terms *webopedia.com*

13. Electronic Research Resources

In addition to the Internet gateways and portals described in section 1, the following sites will assist you in accessing information:

- The American Nurses Association's *Online Journal of Issues in Nursing nursingworld.org/ojin*
- Cumulative Index to Nursing and Allied Health Literature (CINAHL) *cinahl.com*:

  Provides indexes of more than 500 journals from 1982 to present.
- National Library of Medicine *gateway.nlm.nih.gov/gw/Cmd*

  Gateway to the U.S. National Library of Medicine, National Institutes of Health, and Department of Health and Human Services.
- PDA Cortex *PDACortex.com*

14. The Nursing Shortage

- "A Continuing Challenge: The Shortage of Educationally Prepared Nursing Faculty" in the *Online Journal of Nursing Issues* at *nursingworld.org/ojin/topic14/tpc14_3.htm*.
- "Faculty Shortages Intensify Nation's Nursing Deficit" *www.aacn.nche/edu/Publications/issues/IB499WB.htm*.

  A comprehensive discussion of the faculty shortage, including strategies to address it
- Johnson & Johnson's™ Campaign for Nursing's Future *discovernursing.com*
- Nurses for a Healthier Tomorrow *nursesource.org*

15. Men in Nursing

- American Assembly of Men in Nursing *aamn.org*
- Men in American Nursing History *geocities.com/Athens/Forum/6011/index.html*

16. Nurses and September 11th

- "Crisis Theory and Intervention: A Critical Component of Nursing Education." Carla Mariano, Ed.D., R.N., H.N.C., *The Journal of the New York State Nurses Association*, Spring/Summer 2002. *nysna.org*
- "Nurses Share Accounts of 9-11 Aftermath." Susan Trossman, R.N., *The American Nurse*, November/December 2001. *nursingworld.org/tan/01novdec/aftermat.htm*
- "Nurses Share Accounts of 9-11 Aftermath." *The American Nurse*, November/December 2001. *nursingworld.org/tan/01/novdec/aftermat.htm*
- "Nursing at Ground Zero." Maria Gatto, R.N., C.H.P.N., *The Journal of the New York State Nurses Association*, Spring/Summer 2002. *nysna.org*
- "Reflections on September 11, 2001." A collection of poems by Jackie Cataldo, B.S.N., R.N. *The Journal of the New York State Nurses Association*, Spring/Summer 2002. *nysna.org*

- "Through the Eyes of a New Yorker." Lucille Yip, R.N. *The Journal of the New York State Nurses Association*, Spring/Summer 2002. *nysna.org*

- "Volunteering with the Red Cross Family Emergency Relief Services." Carol Noll Hoskins, Ph.D., R.N., F.A.A.N., *The Journal of the New York State Nurses Association*, Spring/Summer 2002. *nysna.org*

- "Nursing at Ground Zero: Experiences During and After September 11th World Trade Center Attack." Suzanne Steffan Dickerson, D.N.S., R.N., Mary Ann Jezewski, Ph.D., R.N., Christine Nelson-Tuttle, M.S., R.N.C., Nancy Shipkey, M.S., R.N., Nancy Wilk, M.S., R.N., and Blythe Crandell, *The Journal of the New York State Nurses Association*, Spring/Summer 2002. *nysna.org*

- For stories about the nine nurses who lost their lives as a result of the attacks on September 11th *geocities.com/heartland/woods/6780*

PEARSON PROFESSIONAL CENTERS OFFERING NCLEX-RN® EXAMINATIONS

The following is a listing of NCLEX-RN® examination sites. More sites will be added in the future. For more information, please visit the website of the National Council of State Boards of Nursing at *ncsbn.org*.

Alabama

600 Vestavia Parkway, Suite 241
Birmingham, AL 35216

AmSouth Bank, Decatur Main
Building
401 Lee Street, Suite 602
Decatur, AL 35602

Carmel Plaza
2623 Montgomery Highway, Suite 4
Dothan, AL 36303

Executive Center I
900 Western America Circle, Suite 504
Mobile, AL 36609

Two East Building
400 East Boulevard, Suite 103
Montgomery, AL 36117

Alaska

Denali Towers North Building
2550 Denali Street, Suite 511
Anchorage, AK 99503

American Samoa

Pago Plaza
P.O. Box AC, Suite 222
Pago Pago, AS 96799

Arizona

555 W. Iron Avenue, Suite 102
Mesa, AZ 85210

The Arizona Business Park
16402 North 28th Avenue
Phoenix, AZ 85053

The Williams Centre
5210 East Williams Circle, Suite 722
Tucson, AZ 85711

Arkansas
John Brown University Center
1401 South Waldron Road, Suite 208
Fort Smith, AR 72903

Benton Building
10802 Executive Center Drive, Suite 201
Little Rock, AR 72211

Landmark Building
210 North State Line, Suite B100
Texarkana, AR 71854

California
Anaheim Corporate Plaza
2190 Towne Center Place, Suite 300
Anaheim, CA 92806

30 River Park Place West, Suite 110
Fresno, CA 93720

South Bay Centre
1515 West 190th Street, Suite 405
Gardena, CA 90248

Broadlake Plaza
360 22nd Street, Suite 502
Oakland, CA 94612-3019

Centrelake Plaza
3401 Centrelake Drive, Suite 675
Ontario, CA 91761

Union Bank Building
70 South Lake Avenue, Suite 780
Pasadena, CA 91101

2190 Larkspur Lane, Suite 400
Redding, CA 96002

3010 Lava Ridge Court, Suite 170
Roseville, CA 95661

9619 Chesapeake Drive, Suite 208
San Diego, CA 92123

Addison Wesley Longman
201 Filbert Street, Suite 200
San Francisco, CA 94133

Koll Lyon Plaza
1641 North First Street, Suite 260
San Jose, CA 95112-4519

Gill Office Building
1010 South Broadway, Suite F
Santa Maria, CA 93454

Westlake Corporate Centre
875 Westlake Boulevard, Suite 106
Westlake Village, CA 91361

Colorado
The Triad
5660 Greenwood Plaza Boulevard,
Suite 510
Greenwood Village, CO 80111

University Center Professional Building
41 Montebello Road, Suite 312
Pueblo CO, 81001

Lake Arbor Plaza
9101 Harlan Street, Suite 320
Westminster, CO 80030

Connecticut
Signature 91
35 Thorpe Avenue
Wallingford, CT 06492

Putnam Park
100 Great Meadow Road, Suite 404
Wethersfield, CT 06109

Delaware
The Kays Building
1012 College Road, Suite 106
Dover, DE 19904

111 Continental Drive, Suite 109
Newark, DE 19713

Florida
Union Street Station
201 SE 2nd Avenue, Suite 208
Gainesville, FL 32601

Corporate Plaza of Deerwood
Building 3
8659 Baypine Road, Suite 305
Jacksonville, FL 32256

1707 Orlando Central Parkway, LLC
1707 Orlando Central Parkway,
Suite 300
Orlando, FL 32809

Kendall I Plaza
8615-8617 South Dixie Highway
Pinecrest, FL 33143

Royal Palm at Southpoint
1000 South Pine Island Road, Suite 260
Plantation, FL 33324

American Bank Building
1777 Tamiami Trail, Suite 508
Port Charlotte, FL 33948

2286-2 Wednesday Street
Tallahassee, FL 32308

Sabal Business Center V
3922 Coconut Palm Drive, Suite 101
Tampa, FL 33619

Georgia
2410 Westgate Boulevard, Suite 102
Albany, GA 31707

The Entrusted Building
3420 Norman Berry Road, Suite 275
Atlanta, GA 30354

Perimeter Center West
1117 Perimeter Center West
Suite W-500
Atlanta, GA 30338

Augusta Riverfront Center
One 10th Street, Suite 665
Augusta, GA 30901

Riverside Corporate Center
4885 Riverside Drive, Suite 101
Macon, GA 31210

Georgetown Center
785 King George Boulevard,
Building 1, Suite C
Savannah, GA 31419

Guam
UIU Building
267 South Marine Drive, Suite 2E
Tamuning, GU 96913

Hawaii
3049 Ualena Street, Suite 406
Honolulu, HI 96819

Hong Kong
Unit 503, 5/F Grand Millennium Plaza
181 Queen's Road, Central
Hong Kong

Idaho
Spectrum View Business Center
1951 South Saturn Way, Suite 200
Boise, ID 83709

Illinois
1 North La Salle Street, Suite 1250
Chicago, IL 60602

103 Airway Drive, Suite 1
Marion, IL 62959

4801 Southwick Drive, Suite 602
Matteson, IL 60443

Norwoods Professional Building
4507 North Sterling Avenue, Suite 302
Peoria IL, 61615

1827 Walden Office Square, Suite 540
Schaumburg, IL 60173

3000 Professional Drive, Suite A
Springfield, IL 62703

Indiana
Eastland Executive Park
4424 Vogel Road, Suite 402
Evansville, IN 47715

Dupont Office Center Building 2
9921 Dupont Circle Drive West, Suite 140
Fort Wayne, IN 46825

Pyramids at College Park
3500 DePauw Boulevard, Suite 2080
Indianapolis, IN 46268

8585 Broadway, Suite 745
Merrillville, IN 46410

630 Wabash Avenue, Suite 221
Terre Haute, IN 47807

Iowa
2441 Coral Court, Suite 2
Coralville, IA 52241

Northwest Bank & Trust Company
100 East Kimberly Road, Suite 401
Davenport, IA 52806

4300 South Lakeport, Suite 204
Sioux City, IA 51106

Colony Park Office Building
3737 Woodland Avenue, Suite 232
West Des Moines, IA 50266

Kansas

Hadley Center
205 East 7th Street, Suite 237
Hays, KS 67601

Gage Office Center Suites
4125 SW Gage Center Drive, Suite 201
Topeka, KS 66604

Equity Financial Center
7701 East Kellogg, Suite 450
Wichita, KS 67207

Kentucky

Alumni Office Park
2317 Alumni Park Plaza, Suite B-130
Lexington, KY 40517

1941 Bishop Lane, Suite 713
Louisville, KY 40218

Louisiana

Corporate Atrium Building
5555 Hilton Avenue, Suite 430
Baton Rouge, LA 70808

Latter Center West
2800 Veterans Boulevard, Suite 215
Metairie, LA 70002

Pierremont Office Park III
920 Pierremont Road, Suite 212
Shreveport, LA 71106

Maine

10 Ridgewood Drive, Suite 2
Bangor ME, 04401

201 Main Street, Suite 4A
Westbrook, ME 04092

Mariana Islands

Del Sol Building
P.O. Box 505140, Garapan, Suite 102
Saipan, MP 96950

Maryland

3108 Lord Baltimore Drive, Suite 103
Baltimore, MD 21244

East-West Towers
4340 East West Highway, Suite 901
Bethesda, MD 20814

Woodmere II
9891 Broken Land Parkway, Suite 108
Columbia, MD 21046

L & F Regional HQ
1315 Mount Herman Road, Suite B
Salisbury MD, 21804

Massachusetts

295 Devonshire Street, Suite 210
Boston, MA 02110

Monarch Place
One Monarch Place, Suite 1110
Springfield, MA 01144

Waltham Office Center
470 Totten Pond Road, 2nd Floor
Waltham, MA 02451

335

Park Office Tower
255 Park Avenue, Suite 604
Worcester, MA 01609

Michigan
Burlington Office Center I
325 E. Eisenhower Parkway, Suite 3A
Ann Arbor, MI 48108

Waters Building
161 Ottawa NW, Suite 307
Grand Rapids, MI 49503

3390 Pine Tree Road, Suite 101
Lansing, MI 48911

Rublein Building
290 Rublein Street, Suite B
Marquette, MI 49855

26555 Evergreen Rd., Suite 822
Southfield, MI 48076

City Center
888 W. Big Beaver Road, Suite 490
Troy, MI 48084

Minnesota
Norman Pointe
5601 Green Valley Drive, Suite 150
Bloomington, MN 55437

Triad Building
7101 Northland Circle, Suite 102
Brooklyn Park, MN 55428

Washington Drive Executive Center
3459 Washington Drive, Suite 107
Eagan, MN 55122-1347

North Shore Bank Place
4815 West Arrowhead Road, Suite 100
Hermantown, MN 55811

Greenview Office Building
1544 Greenview Drive SE, Suite 200
Rochester, MN 55902

Mississippi
Woodlands Office Park
795 Woodlands Parkway, Suite 107
Ridgeland, MS 39157

431 W. Main Street, Suite 340
Tupelo, MS 38801

Missouri
Buttonwood Building
3610 Buttonwood Drive, Suite 102A
Columbia, MO 65201

Ward Parkway Corporate Centre
9200 Ward Parkway, Suite 101
Kansas City, MO 64114

Eleven Eleven Building
1111 South Glenstone, Suite 2-103
Springfield, MO 65804

Center Forty Building
1600 South Brentwood Boulevard,
Suite 120
St. Louis, MO 63144

Montana

Transwestern 1 Building
404 North 31st Street, Suite 230
Billings, MT 59101

Arcade Building
111 N. Last Chance Gulch, Suite 4K
Helena, MT 59601

Nebraska

44 Corporate Place Office Park
300 North 44th Street, Suite 104
Lincoln, NE 68503

Nebraskaland Bank Building
121 North Dewey, Suite 201
North Platte, NE 69101

Omni Corporate Park
10832 Old Mill Road,
Suite 4
Omaha, NE 68154

Nevada

101 Convention Center Drive,
Suite 690
Las Vegas, NV 89109

Corporate Point
5250 South Virginia, Suite 301
Reno, NV 89502

New Hampshire

Capital Plaza
2 Capital Plaza, 4th Floor
Concord, NH 03301

New Jersey

Guarantee Trust Building
1125 Atlantic Avenue, Suite 107
Atlantic City, NJ 08401

1099 Wall Street West, Suite 106
Lyndhurst, NJ 07071

Princeton Forrestal Village
125 Village Boulevard, Suite 302
Princeton, NJ 08540

Pride Building
1543 Route 27
Somerset, NJ 08873

New Mexico

Bank of Albuquerque
2500 Louisiana Boulevard NE,
Suite LL1-B
Albuquerque, NM 87110

New York

1375 Washington Avenue,
Suite 108
Albany, NY 12206

Overpass
45 Main Street, Suite 706
Brooklyn, NY 11201

6700 Kirkville Road, Suite 204
East Syracuse, NY 13057

421-423 East Main Street, Suite 100
Endicott, NY 13760

2950 Expressway Drive South,
Suite 145
Islandia, NY 11749

500 Fifth Avenue, Suite 3120
New York, NY 10110

97-34 64th Road
(97-77 Queens Boulevard)
Rego Park, NY 11374

The Design Center
3445 Winton Place, Suite 238
Rochester, NY 14623

Gardens Office I
1110 South Avenue, Suite 400
Staten Island, NY 10314

122 Business Park Drive, Suite 4
Utica, NY 13502

18564 US Route 11, Suite 7
Watertown, NY 13601

Cross West Office Center
399 Knollwood Road, Suite 218
White Plains, NY 10603

Centerpointe Corporate Park
325 Essjay Road, Suite 104
Williamsville, NY 14221

North Carolina
One Town Square
One Town Square Boulevard, Suite 350
Asheville, NC 28803-5007

Charlotte Park
4601 Charlotte Park Drive, Suite 340
Charlotte, NC 28217

1105-B Corporate Drive, Suite B
Greenville, NC 27858

CEI Building
8024 Glenwood Avenue, Suite 106
Raleigh, NC 27612

Market Street Central
2709 Market Street, Suite 206
Wilmington, NC 28405

Stratford Oaks
514 South Stratford Road, Suite 100
Winston-Salem, NC 27103

North Dakota
Kirkwood Office Tower
919 South 7th Street, Suite 400
Bismarck, ND 58504

Meyer Building
1150 Prairie Parkway, Suite 103
West Fargo, ND 58078

Ohio
Springside Center
231 Springside Drive, Suite 125
Bath, OH 44333

Lakepointe Office
3201 Enterprise Parkway,
Suite 10 Basement
Beachwood, OH 44122

Cornell Plaza
11300 Cornell Park Drive, Suite 140
Cincinnati, OH 45242

355 E. Campus View Boulevard,
Suite 140
Columbus, OH 43235

Imperial Plaza Office Building
1129 Miamisburg-Centerville Road,
Suite 203
Dayton, OH 45449

OffiCenter
700 Taylor Road, Suite 180
Gahanna, OH 43230

Metro Woods Building
1789 Indian Wood Circle, Suite 120
Maumee, OH 43537

Twin Towers
2001 Crocker Road, Suite 350
Westlake, OH 44145

Oklahoma
5100 N. Brookline, Suite 282
Oklahoma City, OK 73112

Town Centre Office Park
Building C
10830 East 45th Street, Suite 210
Tulsa, OK 74146

Oregon
Park Plaza West - Building 3
10700 SW Beaverton Hillsdale Highway,
Suite 595
Beaverton, OR 97005

3560 Excel Drive, Suite 105
Medford, OR 97504

The Mission—17th Building
1660 Oak Street SE, Suite 250
Salem, OR 97301

Pennsylvania
Commerce Corporate Center II
5100 Tighman Street, Suite B-30
Allentown, PA 18104

Edgewood Plaza
3123 West 12th Street, Suite D
Erie, PA 16505

801 East Park Drive, Suite 101
Harrisburg, PA 17111

Pennsylvania Business Campus
110 Gibraltar Road, Suite 227
Horsham, PA 19044

205 Granite Run Drive, Suite 130
Lancaster, PA 17601

1500 Ardmore Boulevard Building
2400 Ardmore Boulevard, Suite 401
Pittsburgh, PA 15221

Penn Center West, Penn Center West II,
Suite 109
Pittsburgh, PA 15276

Stadium Office Park
330 Montage Mountain Rd, Suite 102
Scranton, PA 18507

Valley Forge Office Center
676 E. Swedesfrod Road, Suite 302
Wayne, PA 19087

Puerto Rico
Plaza Scotiabank
273 Ponce de Leon Avenue, Suite 501
San Juan, PR 00917

Rhode Island
Metro Center Boulevard
301 Metro Center Boulevard, Suite 103
Warwick, RI 02886

South Carolina
Westpark Center II
107 Westpark Boulevard, Suite 170
Columbia, SC 29210

Halton Commons Office Park
301-D Halton Road
Greenville, SC 29606

Rivergate Center II
4975 LaCrosse Road, Suite 255
North Charleston, SC 29406

South Dakota
VanBuskirk Office Building
5101 South Nevada Avenue, Suite 130
Sioux Falls, SD 57108

South Korea
Kolon Building, 6th Floor
45 Mukyo-Dong, Chung-Gu
Seoul 100-722
South Korea

Tennessee
Franklin Building
5726 Marlin Road, Suite 310
Chattanooga, TN 37411

Sun Trust Bank Building
207 Mockingbird Lane, Suite 401
Johnson City, TN 37604

Keystone Center
135 Fox Road, Suite C
Knoxville, TN 37922

6060 Poplar Building
6060 Poplar Avenue, Suite LL01
Memphis, TN 38119

Riverview Office Building
545 Mainstream Drive, Suite 410
Nashville, TN 37228

Texas
500 Chestnut, Suite 856
Abilene, TX 79602

1616 S. Kentucky, Suite C305
Amarillo, TX 79102

301 Congress Ave., Suite 565
Ausin, TX 78701

Prosperity Bank Building
6800 West Loop South, Suite 405
Bellaire, TX 77401

Corona South Building
4646 Corona Drive, Suite 175
Corpus Christi, TX 78411

9101 LBJ Freeway, Suite 480
Dallas, TX 75243

Coventry III Building
4445 North Mesa Street, Suite 119
El Paso, TX 79902

8876 Gulf Freeway Building
8876 Gulf Freeway, Suite 220
Houston, TX 77017

500 Grapevine Highway, Suite 401
Hurst, TX 76054-2707

Wells Fargo Tower
1500 Broadway, Suite 1113
Lubbock, TX 79401

Building 4-228
3300 North A Street, Suite 228
Midland, TX 79705-5457

10000 San Pedro, Suite 175
San Antonio, TX 78216

909 East Southeast Loop 323,
Suite 625
Tyler, TX 75701

1105 Wooded Acres, Suite 406
Waco, TX 76710

United Kingdom
190 High Holborn
London WCIV 7BH
United Kingdom

Utah
11734 Election Road, Suite 180
Draper, UT 84020

Business Depot Ogden
1150 South Depot Drive, Suite 130
Ogden, UT 84404

Vermont
30 Kimball, Suite 202
South Burlington, VT 05403

Virginia
424 Graves Mill Road, Building 200,
Suite A
Lynchburg, VA 24502

Two Oyster Point
825 Diligence Drive, Suite 120
Newport News, VA 23606

7202 Glen Forest Drive, Suite 303
Richmond, VA 23226

Northpark Business Center
6701 Peters Creek Road, Suite 108
Roanoke, VA 24019

Centennial Plaza
8391 Old Courthouse Road, Suite 201
Vienna, VA 22182

Virgin Islands
Nisky Center, Suite 730 East Wing
St. Thomas, VI 00802

Washington
Oaksdale Center Building East
1300 S. W. 7th Street, Suite 113
Renton, WA 98055

Mullan Centre
1410 North Mullan, Suite 203
Spokane, WA 99206

1701 Creekside Loop, Suite 110
Yakima, WA 98902

Washington, DC
1615 L Street NW, Suite 410
Washington, DC 20036

West Virginia
BB&T Square
300 Summers Street, Suite 430
Charleston, WV 25301

The Pinion Building
150 Clay Street, Suite 420
Morgantown, WV 26505

Wisconsin
Bishops Woods Center
13555 Bishops Court, Suite L10
Brookfield, WI 53005

3610 Oakwood Mall Drive, Suite 102
Eau Claire, WI 54701

Johnson Bank Building
7500 Green Bay Road, Suite 311
Kenosha, WI 53142

Prairie Trail Office, Suites II
8517 Excelsior Drive, Suite 105
Madison, WI 53717

Wyoming
Aspen Creek
800 Werner Court, Suite 310
Casper, WY 82601

ANCC MAGNET STATUS HEALTH ORGANIZATIONS

Healthcare organizations granted Magnet status have characteristics and outcomes that are positive for clients, nurses, and employers. In these organizations, client satisfaction is high with shorter lengths of stay; nursing satisfaction is high with nurses reporting more control over their nursing practice; employers report lower burnout rates and an enhanced ability to attract and retain nurses. At the time of the publication of this book, the Commission on Magnet Program recognized the following healthcare organizations for their excellence in nursing service:

Aurora Health Care—Metro Region

The system includes the following five facilities:

Auroa Medical Center—
 Washington Country
St. Luke's Medical Center
St. Luke's South Shore
Sinai Aurora Medical Center
West Allis Memorial Hospital
Contact: Regional Nursing Operations
 & Clinical Integration
c/o West Allis Memorial Hospital
8901 West Lincoln Avenue
West Allis, WI 53227
Contact: Karen Fiorelli, R.N., B.S.N.,
 Coordinator for Performance
 Improvement, Center for Nursing
 Research and Practice

Tel: 414-219-3565
Fax: 414-219-3505
Email: karen.fiorelli@aurora.org
aurora.org

Avera McKennan Hospital & University Health Center

800 East 21st Street
P.O. Box 5045
Sioux Falls, SD 57117-5045
Contact: Carla Borchardt, M.S., R.N.,
 B.C., Director Professional Practice,
 Magnet Project Director
Tel: 605-322-7828
Fax: 605-322-1287
Email: carla.borchardt@mckennan.org
mckennan.org

Baptist Hospital

8900 North Kendall Drive
Miami, FL 33176
Contact: Diane Bolton, R.N., Director,
  Acute and Critical Care
Tel: 305-596-6568
Fax: 305-273-2361
Email: dianeb@bhssf.org
baptisthealth.net

Capital Health System

750 Brunswick Avenue
Trenton, NJ 08638
Contact: Patricia Cavanaugh, M.S.N, R.N.,
  Vice President Patient Services/
  Chief Nursing Officer
Tel: 609-394-4000, ext. 4522
Fax: 609-394-4032
Email: pcavanaugh@chsnj.org
Contact: Gail Johnson, Ed.D., M.S.N,
  R.N., CNAA-BC, Magnet Project
  Director/Communicator
Tel: 609-394-6000 ext. 2289
Fax: 609-394-6682
Email: gjohnson@chsnj.org
capitalhealth.org

Catawba Valley Medical Center

810 Fairgrove Church Road, SE
Hickory, NC 28602
Contact: Edward L. Beard, Jr., M.S.N,
  R.N., C.N.A.A., Vice President,
  Patient Care Services
Tel: 828-326-3881
Fax: 828-326-3371
Email: ebeard@catawbavalleymc.org

Contact: Susan Bumgarner, M.S.N,
  R.N.C., C.N.A.A., B.C., Administrator
  Medical/Surgical Nursing Services
Tel: 828-326-2188
Fax: 828-326-3315
Email: sbumgarner@catawbavalleymc.
  org
catawbavalleymc.org

Cedars-Sinai Medical Center

8700 Beverly Boulevard
Los Angeles, CA 90048
Contact: Jane W. Swanson, Ph.D., R.N.,
  C.N.A.A., Director Institute for
  Professional Nursing Development
Tel: 310-423-5185
Fax: 310-423-6179
Email: swansonj@cshs.org
www.cedars-sinai.org

Children's Memorial Medical Center

2300 Children's Plaza
Department of Nursing Administration
Chicago, IL 60614
Contact: Michelle M. Stephenson,
  M.S.N, R.N., Chief Nurse Executive
  Mail Box #5
Tel: 773-880-4106
Contact: Elaine Graf, Ph.D., R.N.,
  P.N.P.,
  Magnet Project Coordinator
  Mail Box #47
Tel: 773-880-4612
Fax: 773-975-8757
Email: egraf@childrensmemorial.org
childrensmemorial.org

East Jefferson General Hospital

4200 Houma Boulevard
Metairie, LA 20006
Contact: Janice Kishner, M.B.A., R.N.,
   Vice President, Nurse Executive
Tel: 504-454-4213
Fax: 504-456-8151
Email: jkishner@ejhospital.com
Contact: Janet Davis, M.P.H., C.H.E.,
   Organizational Effectiveness
   Specialist
Tel: 504-454-4792
Fax: 504-454-5299
Email: jcdavis@ejhospital.com
eastjeffhospital.com

Englewood Hospital & Medical Center

350 Engle Street
Englewood, NJ 07631
Contact: Edna Cadmus, Ph.D., R.N.,
   C.N.A.A.,
   Sr. Vice President, Patient Care
   Services
Tel: 201-894-3199
Fax: 201-894-1345
englewoodhospital.com

Fox Chase Cancer Center

333 Cottman Avenue
Philadelphia, PA 19111
Contact: Anne Jadwin, R.N., M.S.N.,
   A.O.C.N., C.N.A., Director of
   Nursing
Tel: 215-214-1684
Fax: 215-728-3008

Email: AE_Jadwin@fccc.edu
Contact: Joanne M. Hambleton, R.N.,
   M.S.N., C.N.A
Tel: 215-728-3009
Fax: 215-728-3008
Email: JM_hambleton@fccc.edu

Hackensack University Medical Center

Nursing Administration Office
30 Prospect Avenue
Hackensack, NJ 07601
Contact: Mary Ann T. Donohue, Ph.D.,
   R.N., A.P.N., C., Manet Project
   Coordinator
Tel: 201-996-2450
Fax: 201-343-0242
Email: mdonohue@huemed.com
humed.com

High Point Regional Health System

HP-5
601 North Elm Street
High Point, NC 27261
Contact: Tammi Erving Mengel, R.N.,
   M.S.N, C.N.A.A., Administrative
   Director of Nursing
Tel: 336-878-6000
Fax: 336-878-6250
Email: tmengel@hprhs.com
Contact: Martha Barham, R.N., M.S.N,
   C.N.A.A., Vice President Inpatient
   Administration, Chief Nursing
   Officer

Tel: 336-878-6000
Fax: 336-878-6250
Email: mbarham@hprhs.com
highpointregional.com

Inova Fairfax Hospital

3300 Gallows Road
Falls Church, VA 22042
Contact: Toni R. Ardabell, R.N., M.S.N.,
   M.B.A., V.P., I.H.S., C.O.O., I.F.H./
   I.F.H.C./I.V.H.I., Interim C.N.E.
Tel: 703-776-3561
Fax: 703-776-3623
Email: Toni.Ardabell@inova.com
Contact: Lorna M. Facteau, R.N.,
   D.N.S.c., Sr. Director Childrens
   Services, I.F.H.C., Behavioral
   Services, I.F.H.
Tel: 703-776-6003
Fax: 703-776-6078
Email: Lorna.Facteau@inova.com
Contact: Diane Yantus, RN, MSN,
   Director, Special Projects
Tel: 703-776-6036
Fax: 703-776-2096
Email: Diane.Yantus@inova.com
inova.com

James A. Haley Veterans' Hospital

Department of Veterans Affairs
13000 Bruce B. Downs Boulevard
Code 118
Tampa, FL 33612
Contact: Sandra K. Janzen, R.N., M.S.,
   C.N.A.A., Chief Nurse Executive,
   Associate Chief of Staff/Nursing

Tel: 813-979-3654
Fax: 813-978-5974
Email: sandra.janzen@med.va.gov
Contact: Susan V. White, Ph.D., R.N.,
   C.P.H.Q., F.N.A.H.Q., Associate
   Chief Nurse/Quality Improvement
Tel: 813-972-2000, ext. 7953
Fax: 813-979-5974
Email: susan.white4@med.va.gov

Jersey Shore Medical Center

1945 Route 33
Neptune, NJ 07754
Contact: Richard Hader, R.N., Ph.D.,
   F.A.A.N., C.H.E.,C.N.A., C.P.H.Q.,
   Senior Vice President, Chief Nursing
   Officer
Tel: 732-776-4632
Fax: 732-776-4731
Email: rhader@meridianhealth.com
Contact: Nancy Shafer-Winter, Senior
   Manager, Patient Care Services
Tel: 732-776-4833
Fax: 732-776-4873
Email: nwinter@meridianhealth.com
Contact: Jane Bliss-Holtz, .D.N.S.c.,
   B.C., Nurse Researcher, Ann May
   Center
Tel: 732-776-2495
jsmc.com

Jewish Hospital

200 Abraham Flexner Way
Louisville, KY 40202
Contact: Lisa Dolan, R.N., M.S.N.,
   C.N.A.,B.C., Interim C.N.O.

Tel: 502-587-4411
Fax: 502-560-8437
Email: lisa.dolan@jhhs.org
Contact:Sherill Cronin, R.N., Ph.D.,
    Nurse Researcher
Tel: 502-587-4192
Fax: 502-560-8437
Email:sherill.cronin@jhhs.org
jewishhospital.org

Kimball Medical Center

600 River Avenue
Lakewood, NJ 08701
Contact: Mary Pat Sullivan, Vice
    President for Patient Care Services
Tel: 732-886-4615
Fax: 732-886-4529
Email: msullivan@sbhcs.com
Contact: Anne Marie Williams, R.N.,
    M.S.N., A.P.N.C., C.E.N.,
Nursing Quality Coordinator
Email: anwilliams@sbhcs.com
sbhcs.com/hospitals/kimbal_medical

Mayo Clinic College of Medicine

200 First Street, S.W.
Rochester, MN 55905
Contact: Debra M. Berland, R.N.,
    Nursing Administrative Specialist,
    Department of Nursing
Tel: 507-255-8690
Fax: 507-255-8873
Email: berland.debra@mayo.edu
mayo.edu

The Methodist Hospital

6565 Fannin M.S.-D793
Houston, TX 77080
Contact: Ann Scanlon McGinity,
    Ph.D., R.N.,
    Vice President, Operation
Tel: 713-441-2332
Email: ascanlon@tmh.tmc.edu
Contact: Mary Shepherd, M.S.N., R.N.,
    C.N.A.A., Magnet Project Director
Tel: 713-441-2531
Fax: 713-441-4427
Email: MLShepherd@tmh.tmc.edu
methodisthealth.com

Middlesex Hospital

28 Crescent Street
Middletown, CT 06457
Contact: Colleen O. Smith, R.N.,
    M.S.N, C.N.A., Vice President for
    Nursing
Tel: 860-344-6460
Fax: 860-344-6779
Email: colleen_smith@midhosp.org
Contact: Kathleen M. Stolzenberger,
    M.S., R.N., Director of Program
    Development
Tel: 860-344-6460
Fax: 860-344-6779
Email: kathleen_stolzenberger@
    midhosp.org
www.midhosp.org

The Miriam Hospital

164 Summit Avenue
Providence, RI 02906
Contact: Rebecca Burke, R.N., M.S.,
    Senior Vice President for Patient
    Care Services, Chief Nursing Officer
Tel: 401-793-3600
Fax: 401-793-3636
Email: rburke@lifespan.org
Contact: Maria Ducharme, M.S., R.N.
    C.N.A-B.C., Magnet Coordinator
Tel: 401-793-3632
Fax: 401-793-3636
Email: mducharm@lifespan.org
lifespan.org

Morristown Memorial Hospital

100 Madison Avenue, Box #23
Morristown, NJ 07962-1956
Contact: Trish O'Keefe, R.N., M.S.N.,
    C.N.A., Chief Nursing Officer
Tel: 973-971-5835
Fax: 973-290-7010
Email: trish.o'keefe@ahsys.org
Contact: Charlotte Qualls, R.N., M.A.,
    Manager Magnet/Shared Governance
Tel: 973-971-5452
Email: charlotte.qualls@ahsys.org
atlantichealth.org/cons

North Carolina Baptist Hospital of Wake Forest University

Baptist Medical Center
Medical Center Boulevard
Winston-Salem, NC 27157
Contact: Barbara C. Smith, M.S.N.,
    R.N., B.C., CNAA, Magnet Project
    Director

Tel: 336-716-4509
Fax: 336-716-5399
Email: barsmith@wfubmc.edu
Contact: A. Patricia Johnson, R.N.,
    M.A. Ed, Vice President, Operations,
    C.N.O.
Tel: 336-716-3424
Fax: 336-716-2067
wfubmc.edu

Poudre Valley Health System, Poudre Valley Hospital

1024 Lemay Avenue
Fort Collins, CO 80524
Contact: Craig Luzinski, R.N., M.S.N.,
    C.N.O.
Tel: 970-495-7141
Email: ddp@pvhs.org
pvhs.org

Providence St. Vincent Medical Center

9205 S.W. Barnes Road
Portland, OR 97225
Contact: Gladys Campbell, R.N.,
    M.S.N.,
    Assistant Administrator Nursing and
    Patient Care
Contact: Traci Hoiting, R.N., M.S.,
    A.C.N.P.-B.C., Director of Nursing
    Education and Quality
Tel: 503-216-2319
Fax: 503-216-0235
Email: traci.hoiting@providence.org
providence.org

Riverview Medical Center

One Riverview Plaza
Red Bank, NJ 07701
Contact: Mary Ellen Strozak, M.S.,
R.N., C.C.R.N., C.N.S., Clinical
Nurse Specialist
Tel: 732-741-2700, ext. 4180
Fax: 732-224-7257
Email: mstrozak@meridianhealth.com
www.meridianhealth.com

Robert Wood Johnson University Hospital

1 Robert Wood Johnson Place
New Brunswick, NJ 08903-2601
Contact: Kathi Sengin, Ph.D., R.N.,
C.N.A.A., Senior Vice President,
Nursing and Patient Services
Tel: 732-937-8874
Fax: 732-937-8699
Email: kathi.sengin@rwjuh.edu
Contact: Anne Bernard, M.S.N., R.N.,
C.P.H.Q., Director of Performance
Improvement and Regulatory
Compliance
Tel: 732-418-8231
Fax: 732-418-8416
Email: Anne.Bernard@rwjuh.edu
rwjuh.edu

Rush University Medical Center

1653 West Congress Parkway
Chicago, IL 60612
Contact: Jane Llewellyn, D.N.S.c., R.N.,
C.N.A.A., Chief Nursing Officer
Contact: Beverly Hancock, M.S., R.N.
Education, Quality Coordinator

Tel: 312-942-8724
Fax: 312-942-3386
Email: Beverly_Hancock@rush.edu
rush.edu

St. Francis Medical Center

601 Hamilton Avenue
Trenton, NJ 08629
Contact: Judy Rottkamp, Assistant Vice
President of Nursing
Tel: 609-599-5759
Fax: 609-599-5779
Email: jrottkamp@CHE-East.org
Contact: Carol McAloon, VP Patient
Care Services/CNO
Tel: 609-599-5283
Fax: 609-599-5779
Email: cmcaloon@CHE-East.org
sfmc.net

St. Joseph's/Candler

5353 Reynolds Street
Savannah, GA 31405
Contact: Sherry Danello, M.S.N., R.N.,
C.N.A.A., Vice President, Patient
Care Services and Chief Nursing
Officer
Tel: 912-819-6640
Fax: 912-691-9049
Email: danellos@sjchs.org
Contact: Susan Howell, Ed.D., R.N.,
A.O.C.N., Director of Professional
Practice
Tel: 912-819-8142
Fax: 912-691-9080
Email: howells@sjchs.org
sjchs.org

Saint Joseph's Hospital of Atlanta

5665 Peachtree Dunwoody Road, N.E.
Atlanta, GA 30342
Contact: Vickie Moore, M.S.N., R.N.,
C.H.E., C.N.A.A.-B.C., Senior Vice
President, Operations
Tel: 404-851-7120
Fax: 404-851-7339
Email: vmoore@sjha.org
Contact: Polly H. Willis, R.N., M.S.N.,
Director, Pulmonary/Renal Services/
Magnet Coordinator
Tel: 404-851-7008
Email: pwillis@sjha.org
stjosephsatlanta.org

Saint Joseph's Regional Medical Center

703 Main Street
Paterson, NJ 07503
Contact: Maria Brennan, R.N., M.S.N.,
C.N.O.
Tel: 973-754-2055
Fax: 973-754-2044
Email: brennanm@sjhmc.org
Contact: Mary Ann Hozak, R.N.,
B.S.N., C.C.R.N., Magnet Project
Director/Communicator
Tel: 973-754-3421
Email: hozakm@sjhmc.org
www.sjhmc.org

St. Luke's Episcopal Hospital

6720 Bertner Avenue
Houston, TX 77030
Contact: Karen Myers, M.S.N., R.N.,
C.N.A.A., B.C., Vice President and
Chief Nursing Officer
Tel: 832-355-4037
Fax: 832-355-6182
Email: kmyers@sleh.com
Contact: Cheryl Lindy, M.S., R.N.,
B.C., C.N.A.A., Director, Nursing &
Patient Education
Tel: 832-355-4458
Fax: 832-355-3019
Email: clindy@sleh.com
sleh.com/sleh

St. Luke's Regional Medical Center

190 E. Bannock Street
Boise, ID 83712
Contact: Noreen Davis, Senior Vice
President, Nursing & Patient Care
Services
Tel: 208-381-2550
Fax: 208-381-2861
Email: davisn@slrmc.org
Contact: Beth Gray, Clinical Director,
Evidence-Based Practice
Tel: 208-381-4292
Fax: 208-381-2564
Email: grayb@slrmc.org
slrmc.org

St. Mary's Hospital Medical Center

707 S. Mills Street
Madison, WI 53715
Contact: Christine Baker, Ph.D.,
R.N., A.P.R.N., B.C., Clinical Nurse
Specialist for Nursing Outcomes
Tel: 608-259-5855
Fax: 608-259-5327
Email: christine_baker@ssmhc.com
Contact: Joan Ellis Beglinger, M.S.N,
M.B.A., R.N., F.A.C.H.E., Vice
President for Patient Services
Tel: 608-258-6735
Fax: 608-259-5327
Email: joan_beglinger@ssmhc.com
stmarysmadison.com

St. Peter's University Hospital

254 Easton Avenue
P.O. Box 591
New Brunswick, NJ 08903-0591
Contact: Kathleen Russell-Babin,
R.N., M.S.N., C.N.A.A., A.P.R.N.-
B.C., Vice President of Patient Care
Services
Tel: 732-745-8600, ext. 8318
Fax: 732-745-7938
Email: krussell-babin@saintpetersuh.
com
Contact: Wendy Silverstein, M.A.,
A.P.R.N.-B.C., Magnet Project
Director/Communicator
Tel: 732-745-8000, ext. 8718
Fax: 732-745-7938
Email: wsilver@saintpetersuh.com
saintpetersuh.com

Southwestern Vermont Medical Center

100 Hospital Drive
Bennington, VT 05201
Contact: Katherine Riley, B.S.N., R.N.,
Director of Women's & Children's
Services
Tel: 802-447-5110
Fax: 802-442-8331
Email: kaf@phin.org
svhealthcare.org

UAB Hospital

1813 Sixth Avenue South
Birmingham, AL 35249-6559
Contact: Cynthia Barginere, Chief
Nursing Officer, M.S.N., R.N.,
Associate Vice Presient
Tel: 205-975-9051
Fax: 205-975-7837
Email: cbarginer@health.uabmc.edu
Contact: Douglas Oliver, M.S.N., R.N.,
Magnet Project Coordinator, C.N.S.
Tel: 205-934-9519
Fax: 205-975-6045
Email: doliver@uabmc.edu
health.uab.edu

University of Colorado Hospital

4200 East Ninth Avenue
Campus Box A020
Denver, CO 80262
Contact: Kathy Smith, M.S., R.N.,
Informatic Nurse Specialist, Magnet
Project Director/ Communicator
Tel: 303-372-5553

Fax: 303-372-5559
Email: kathy.smith@uch.edu
Contact: Colleen Goode, Ph.D., R.N.,
     F.A.A.N., Vice President Patient
     Services and Chief Nursing Officer
Tel: 303-372-5379
Fax: 303-372-5385
Email: colleen.goode@uch.edu
www.uch.edu

University of Kentucky Hospital

800 Rose Street
Lexington, KY 40536
Contact: Karen Stefaniak, Ph.D., R.N.,
     Associate Director/Chief Nursing
     Officer
Tel: 859-323-5982
Fax: 859-323-2044
Email: kastef00@uky.edu
Contact: Patricia Powers, M.S.N.,
     R.N., Director of Nursing
     Practice/Support Services/ Magnet
     Coordinator
Tel: 859-323-5330
Fax: 859-323-9923
Email: phpower@uky.edu
www.mc.uky.edu

The University of Texas M.D. Anderson Cancer Center

1515 Holcombe Boulevard
Houston, TX 77030-4098
Contact: Barbara L. Summers, Ph.D.,
     R.N., Vice President, Chief Nursing
     Officer and Head, Division of
     Nursing
Tel: 713-792-7475

Fax: 713-792-0795
Email: bsummers@mdanderson.org
Contact: Harriett Chaney, Ph.D.,
     A.P.R.N.-B.C., Director Nursing
     Programs
Tel: 713-792-7104
Fax: 713-794-4917
Email: hchaney@mdanderson.org
mdanderson.org

University of Washington Medical Center

Box 356153
Seattle, WA 98195-6153
Contact: Catherine Broom, A.P.R.N.,
     C.N.S., Magnet Project Coordinator
Tel: 206-598-4627
Fax: 206-598-6576
Email: bosley@u.washington.edu
www.uwmedicine.org

STATE BOARDS OF NURSING AND LICENSING REQUIREMENTS*

Alabama

Board of Nursing
RSA Plaza, Suite 250
P.O. Box 303900
770 Washington Avenue
Montgomery, AL 36130-3900
Phone: 334-242-4060
Fax: 334-242-4360
abn.state.al.us/
Temporary Permit: 90 days by exam; three months if by endorsement; $50
State Board Fee: $85
Additional State Endorsement: $85
NCLEX-RN* Test Fee: $200
Re-Examination Limitations: Every 91 days; $85
License Renewal: December 31, per biennial renewal period; $75
CEU Requirements: 24 contact hours per biennial renewal period. Nurses licensed by examination are required to have four contact hours of Board-provided continuing education for the first renewal (included in the total number of hours to be earned). MEDCEU contact hours are no longer accepted.

Alaska

Board of Nursing
Dept. of Community and Economic Development
Division of Occupational Licensing
P.O. Box 110806
333 Willoughby Avenue, 9th Floor
Juneau, AK 99811-0806
Phone: 907-465-2544 (last names A–K);
    907-465-2648 (last names L–Z)
Fax: 907-465-2974
dced.state.ak.us/occ/pnur.htm
Temporary Permit: Four months by exam or by endorsement; $50
State Board Fee: $215 permanent license fee; $50 application fee plus $59 fingerprint fee
Additional State Endorsement: $215 permanent license fee; $50 application fee plus $59 fingerprint fee
NCLEX-RN* Test Fee: $200
Re-Examination Limitations: Every 91 days. Must pass within five years, then retake with remediation.
License Renewal: November 30, every even year; $215

*The information in this section is up-to-date at the time of publication. However, state licensing requirements may change after this book is published. Contact your state licensure board for the latest information.

CEU Requirements: Method 1: Two of the three required for renewal: (1) 30 contact hours of CE, (2) 30 hours of professional nursing activities, (3) 320 hours of nursing employment. Method 2: Completed a board-approved nursing refresher course. Method 3: Attained a degree or certificate in nursing, beyond the requirements of the original license, by successfully completing at least two required courses. Method 4: Successfully completed the National Council Licensing Examination.

Arizona

Arizona State Board of Nursing
4747 N. 7th Street, Suite 200
Phoenix, AZ 85014
Phone: 602-889-5150
Fax: 602-889-5155
www.azbn.gov
Temporary Permit: Four months pending results of fingerprint check, must have already passed the exam; $25
State Board Fee: $220, plus $43 fingerprint fee
Additional State Endorsement: $150, plus $43 fingerprint fee
NCLEX-RN* Test Fee: $200
Re-Examination Limitations: Every 45 days; $60
License Renewal: June 30, every four years; $120
CEU Requirements: None

Arkansas

State Board of Nursing
University Tower Building
1123 South University, Suite 800
Little Rock, AR 72204-1619
Phone: 501-686-2700
Fax: 501-686-2714
www.arsbn.org
Temporary Permit: Up to 90 days if by endorsement; $25
State Board Fee: $75
Additional State Endorsement: $100
NCLEX-RN* Test Fee: $200
Re-Examination Limitations: Every 91 days
License Renewal: Birthday, every two years; $75
CEU Requirements: Licensees who hold an active nursing license shall document completion of one of the following during each renewal period:
a. Fifteen (15) practice focused contact hours from a nationally recognized or state continuing education approval body recognized by the ASBN; or
b. Certification or re-certification during the renewal period by a national certifying body recognized by the ASBN; or
c. An academic course in nursing or related field; and
d. Provide other evidence as requested by the Board.

California

Board of Registered Nursing
1625 North Market Blvd, Suite N217
Sacramento, CA 95834
Phone: 916-574-8637
Fax: 916-327-4402
rn.ca.gov
Temporary Permit: Interim license pending results of first exam; six months if by endorsement; $30
State Board Fee: $75 application fee, plus $32 fingerprint fee
Additional State Endorsement: $50, plus $56 fingerprint fee
NCLEX-RN® Test Fee: $200
Re-Examination Limitations: Every 91 days; $75
License Renewal: Last day of the month following birth month, every two years; $85
CEU Requirements: 30 contact hours every two years.

Colorado

Board of Nursing
1560 Broadway, Suite 880
Denver, CO 80202
Phone: 303-894-2430
Fax: 303-894-2821
dora.state.co.us/nursing/
Temporary Permit: 90 days; four months if by endorsement. Fee is included in application fee.
State Board Fee: $83 initial exam
Additional State Endorsement: $38
NCLEX-RN® Test Fee: $200
Re-Examination Limitations: Every 91 days; $75

License Renewal: September 30, every two years; $93
CEU Requirements: None

Connecticut

Board of Examiners for Nursing
Department of Public Health
RN Licensure
410 Capitol Avenue
MS# 12 APP
P.O. Box 340308
Hartford, CT 06134-0308
Phone: 860-509-7603
Fax: 860-509-8457
www. dph.state.ct.us/licensure/ licensure.htm#R
Temporary Permit: 90 days from completion of nursing program. Temporary permit also available for endorsement applicants, valid for 120 days, nonrenewable; must hold valid license in another state. Fee is included in application fee.
State Board Fee: $90
Additional State Endorsement: $90
NCLEX-RN® Test Fee: $200
Re-Examination Limitations: Every 91 days, no more than four times in one year
License Renewal: Last day of birth month, every year; $50
CEU Requirements: None

Delaware

Division of Professional Regulation
Board of Nursing
861 Silver Lake Boulevard
Cannon Building, Suite 203
Dover, DE 19904-2467

Phone: 302-744-4516
Fax: 302-739-2711
professionallicensing.state.de.us/boards/
nursing/index.shtml
Temporary Permit: 90 days by
endorsement or pending results of first
exam; $25–$30
State Board Fee: $77
Additional State Endorsement: $52–
$16
NCLEX-RN° Test Fee: $200
Re-examination Limitations: Every 46
days; $10. Re-examination can occur no
sooner than 45 calendar days after the
previous exam.
License Renewal: Renewal applications
are mailed to all active licensees
approximately ten weeks before the
expiration date of their current license.
You are notified of the amount of the
renewal fee at the time of renewal.
License Renewal: February 28, May 31,
and September 30, every odd year; $67
CEU Requirements: 30 contact hours
every two years. Nurses licensed by
exam are exempt from CE requirements
for the first renewal after initial licensure.
Minimum practice requirement of
1,000 hours in five years or 400 hours
in two years.

District of Columbia

Department of Health
Board of Nursing
717 14th Street, NW, Suite 600
Washington, DC 20005
Phone: 877-672-2174
Fax: 202-727-8471
hpla.doh.dc.gov/hpla/site/default.asp

Temporary Permit: None
State Board Fee: $78 license fee; $65
application fee
Additional State Endorsement: $111
license fee; $65 application fee
NCLEX-RN° Test Fee: $200
Re-Examination Limitations: Every 91
days; $65
License Renewal: June 30, every two
years; $111
CEU Requirements: The completion
of twenty-four (24) contact hours of
continuing education in the licensee's
current area of practice is required
commencing with the renewal period
of 2006.

Florida

Board of Nursing
4052 Bald Cypress Way, BIN C02
Tallahassee, FL 32399
Phone: 850-245-4125
Fax: 850-245-4172
www.doh.state.fl.us/mqa/nursing/
Temporary Permit: 90 days pending
results of first exam; 60 days if by
endorsement. Fee is included in
licensure fee.
State Board Fee: $190 initial exam
Additional State Endorsement: $212
NCLEX-RN° Test Fee: $200
Re-Examination Limitations: Every
45 days; remedial training program is
required after three attempts; $105
License Renewal: Every odd year; $65
CEU Requirements: 25 contact hours
every two years. One hour per month.
Two hours in the prevention of medical
errors and one hour each in HIV and

domestic violence by a provider approved by the state of Florida; proof of training in latter two prior to licensure. Nurses licensed by examination are exempt from CE requirements in the period following first licensure.

Georgia
Board of Nursing
237 Coliseum Drive
Macon, GA 31217-3858
Phone: 478-207-1300
Fax: 478-207-1363
sos.state.ga.us/plb/rn
Temporary Permit: Six months if by endorsement. Fee is included in application fee.
State Board Fee: $40
Additional State Endorsement: $60
NCLEX-RN® Test Fee: $200, plus $12 when registering by telephone
Re-Examination Limitations: Every 91 days, three years maximum
License Renewal: January 31, every even year; $65
CEU Requirements: None

Hawaii
DCCA—PVL
Board of Nursing
P.O. Box 3469
Honolulu, HI 96801
Phone: 808-586-3000
Fax: 808-586-2689
hawaii.gov.dcca/areas/pvl/boards/nursing
Temporary Permit: By endorsement with employment verification
State Board Fee: $40

Additional State Endorsement:
$135 or $180, depending on the year license is issued. Noted on application information sheet.
NCLEX-RN® Test Fee: $200
Re-Examination Limitations: Every 91 days
License Renewal: June 30, every odd year (deadline May 31); $90
CEU Requirements: None

Idaho
Board of Nursing
280 North 8th Street, Suite 210
P.O. Box 83720
Boise, ID 83720-0061
Phone: 208-334-3110
Fax: 208-334-3262
www2.state.id.us/ibn/ibnhome.htm
Temporary Permit: 90 days if by endorsement, $115
State Board Fee: $90, plus $34 fingerprint fee
Additional State Endorsement: $110, plus $34 fingerprint fee
NCLEX-RN® Test Fee: $200
Re-Examination Limitations: Every 91 days
License Renewal: August 31, every odd year; $50
CEU Requirements: None

Illinois
Department of Professional Regulation
320 W. Washington Street, 3rd Floor
Springfield, IL 62786
Phone: 217-785-0800
Fax: 217-782-7645
www. idfpr.com/dpr/WHO/nurs.asp

357

Temporary Permit: Three-month approval letter by examination; six months by endorsement; $25
State Board Fee: $50
Additional State Endorsement: $50
NCLEX-RN˚ Test Fee: $200
Re-Examination Limitations: Every 91 days, three years from first writing to board
License Renewal: May 31, every even year; $30
CEU Requirements: None

Indiana

State Board of Nursing
Professional Licensing Agency
402 West Washington Street, Room W072
Indianapolis, IN 46204
Phone: 317-234-2043
Fax: 317-233-4236
state.in.us/hpb/boards/isbn
Temporary Permit: 90 days if by endorsement; $10
State Board Fee: $50
Additional State Endorsement: $50
NCLEX-RN˚ Test Fee: $200
Re-Examination Limitations: Every 91 days
License Renewal: October 31, every odd year; $50
CEU Requirements: None

Iowa

Board of Nursing
Riverpoint Business Park
400 SW 8th Street, Suite B
Des Moines, IA 50309-4685
Phone: 515-281-3255
Fax: 515-281-4825
www.state.ia.us/government/nursing
Temporary Permit: 30 days if by endorsement. Fee is included in application fee.
State Board Fee: $93, plus $50 criminal history background check
Additional State Endorsement: $119, plus $50 criminal history background check
NCLEX-RN˚ Test Fee: $200
Re-Examination Limitations: Every 91 days
License Renewal: 30 days prior to the 15th of month of birth, every three years; $99
CEU Requirements: 36 contact hours or 3.6 CEUs every three years

Kansas

State Board of Nursing
Landon State Office Building
900 SW Jackson, Suite 1051
Topeka, KS 66612-1230
Phone: 785-296-4929
Fax: 785-296-3929
ksbn.org
Temporary Permit: Pending results of first exam, or no longer than 90 days from graduation; 120 days if by endorsement. Fee is included in application fee.

State Board Fee: $75
Additional State Endorsement: $75
NCLEX-RN* Test Fee: $200
Re-Examination Limitations: Every 91 days, unlimited number of times; after two years the applicant must provide an approved study plan
License Renewal: Month of birth, every two years; $60
CEU Requirements: 30 contact hours every two years

Kentucky

Board of Nursing
312 Whittington Parkway, Suite 300
Louisville, KY 40222-5172
Phone: 502-429-3300
Fax: 502-429-3311
kbn.ky.gov
Temporary Permit: No temporary work permits are issued to new graduates. Six months by endorsement. Fee included in application fee.
State Board Fee: $110
Additional State Endorsement: $150
NCLEX-RN* Test Fee: $200
Re-Examination Limitations: Every 46 days
License Renewal: October 31, every even year; $105. Beginning in July 2006, annual; $50.
CEU Requirements: 14 contact hours or equivalent every year, plus two hours of mandatory HIV/AIDS CE to be earned within the appropriate 10-year period. A one-time, three-hour domestic violence requirement must be completed within three years of the date of initial licensing.

Louisiana

Board of Nursing
5207 Essen Lane, Suite 6
Baton Rouge, LA 70809
Phone: 225-763-3570
Fax: 225-763-3580
www.lsbn.state.la.us
Temporary Permit: Pending results of first exam; 90 days if by endorsement. Fee is included in application fee. Permit becomes void when exam results received.
State Board Fee: $100, plus $50 fingerprint fee
Additional State Endorsement: $100
NCLEX-RN* Test Fee: $200
Re-Examination Limitations: Every 91 days, up to four times
License Renewal: January 31, every year; $45
CEU Requirements: For all RNs: 5, 10, or 15 contact hours every year, based on employment

Maine

Board of Nursing
161 Capitol Street
158 State House Station
Augusta, ME 04333
Phone: 207-287-1133
Fax: 207-287-1149
www.state.me.us/boardofnursing
Temporary Permit: 90 days. Fee is included in application fee.
State Board Fee: $60
Additional State Endorsement: $60
NCLEX-RN* Test Fee: $200
Re-Examination Limitations: Every 91 days

License Renewal: Birthday, every two years; $40
CEU Requirements: None

Maryland

Board of Nursing
4140 Patterson Avenue
Baltimore, MD 21215-2254
Phone: 410-585-1900
Fax: 410-358-3530
mbon.org
Temporary Permit: 90 days by endorsement, not renewable; $25
State Board Fee: $75
Additional State Endorsement: $75
NCLEX-RN° Test Fee: $200
Re-Examination Limitations: Every 46 days
License Renewal: 28th day of month of birth, every year; $60.25
CEU Requirements: None

Massachusetts

Division of Professional Licensure
Board of Registration in Nursing
239 Causeway Street, Suite 200
2nd Floor
Boston, MA 02114
Phone: 617-973-0800
Fax: 617-973-0984
www.state.ma.us/reg/boards/rn/
Temporary Permit: Not granted
State Board Fee: $375, includes test fee
Additional State Endorsement: $130
NCLEX-RN° Test Fee: $200, included in state board fee
Re-Examination Limitations: Every 91 days; $75

License Renewal: Birthday, every even year; $80
CEU Requirements: 15 contact hours every two years

Michigan

Bureau of Health Professions
Michigan Department of Community Health
Board of Nursing
Ottawa Building
611 West Ottawa, 1st Floor
Lansing, MI 48933
Physical Address:
Bureau of Health Professions
Ottawa Building
611 W. Ottawa Street, 1st Floor
Lansing, MI 48933
Mailing Address:
Bureau of Health Professions
P.O. Box 30670
Lansing, MI 48909-8170
Phone: 517-335-0918
Fax: 517-373-2179
michigan.gov/mdch/
Temporary Permit: No longer available
State Board Fee: $48
Additional State Endorsement: $48
NCLEX-RN° Test Fee: $200
Re-Examination Limitations: Every 91 days, up to six attempts within three years. Must pass exam within six months of first attempt or attend another RN education program.
License Renewal: March 31, every two years; $48
CEU Requirements: 25 credits every two years

Minnesota

Board of Nursing
2829 University Avenue, SE #200
Minneapolis, MN 55414-3253
Phone: 612-617-2270
Fax: 612-617-2190
www.nursingboard.state.mn.us/
Temporary Permit: 60 days, license by exam; $60. One year if by endorsement, no fee.
State Board Fee: $105 initial exam
Additional State Endorsement: $105
NCLEX-RN® Test Fee: $200
Re-Examination Limitations: Every 91 days. Must retake within one year or application becomes null; $60.
License Renewal: Birth month, every two years; $85
CEU Requirements: 24 contact hours every two years

Mississippi

Board of Nursing
1935 Lakeland Drive, Suite B
Jackson, MS 39216
Phone: 601-944-4826
Fax: 601-364-2352
www.msbn.state.ms.us/
Temporary Permit: 90 days by endorsement; $25
State Board Fee: $60
Additional State Endorsement: $60
NCLEX-RN® Test Fee: $200
Re-Examination Limitations: Every 91 days
License Renewal: December 31, every even year; $50
CEU Requirements: None

Missouri

Board of Nursing
3605 Missouri Boulevard
P.O. Box 656
Jefferson City, MO 65102-0656
Phone: 573-751-0681
Fax: 573-751-0075
www.pr.mo.gov/nursing.asp
Temporary Permit: Six months. Fee is included in application fee.
State Board Fee: $45 initial exam
Additional State Endorsement: $55
NCLEX-RN® Test Fee: $200
Re-Examination Limitations: Every 91 days; $40
License Renewal: April 30, every odd year; $80 (plus additional fee for renewing online).
CEU Requirements: None

Montana

Department of Labor and Industry
Board of Nursing
301 South Park, Room 430
P.O. Box 200513
Helena, MT 59620-0513
Phone: 406-841-2340
Fax: 406-841-2343
*mt.gov/dli/bsd/license/bsd_boards/
nur_board/board_page.asp*
Temporary Permit: 90 days by endorsement or exam; $25
State Board Fee: $100
Additional State Endorsement: $200
NCLEX-RN® Test Fee: $200
Re-Examination Limitations: Every 91 days, up to five attempts in three years. After failing twice, must present a plan of study to the Board before

next retake. If one doesn't pass within three years, must take Nursing Program before sixth retake.
License Renewal: December 31, every two years; $100
CEU Requirements: None

Nebraska
Department of HHS Regulation and Licensure
Nursing and Nursing Support Section
State Office Building
301 Centennial Mall South, 3rd Floor
P.O. Box 94986
Lincoln, NE 68509-4986
Phone: 402-471-4376
Fax: 402-471-1066
www.hhs.state.ne.us/crl/nursing/Rn-Lpn/rn-lpn.htm
Temporary Permit: 60 days if by endorsement. Fee is included in licensing fee.
State Board Fee: $75 plus $2 LAP fee
Additional State Endorsement: $75 plus $2 LAP fee
NCLEX-RN* Test Fee: $200
Re-Examination Limitations: Every 91 days
License Renewal: October 31, every even year; $75 plus $2 LAP fee. If 90 days prior to expiration, $10
CEU Requirements: 20 contact hours every two years with 500 practice hours every five years, or a refresher course of study in previous five years. New graduates are exempt from CEU requirements for the first renewal period for two years from graduation.

Nevada
Board of Nursing
2500 W. Sahara Avenue, Suite 207
Las Vegas, NV 89102-4392
Phone: 702-486-5800 or 888-590-6726
Fax: 702-486-5803
nursingboard.state.nv.us/
Temporary License: Four months, not renewable. Fee is included in application fee; $50 if not seeking permanent license.
State Board Fee: $100
Additional State Endorsement: $105
NCLEX-RN* Test Fee: $200
Re-Examination Limitations: Every 91 days, up to three times, then only with remediation
License Renewal: Birthday, every two years; $100
CEU Requirements: 30 contact hours every two years at renewal. New grads may be exempt from CE requirements for their first renewal period.

New Hampshire
Board of Nursing
21 South Fruit Street, Suite 16
Concord, NH 03301-2431
Phone: 603-271-2323
Fax: 603-271-6605
state.nh.us/nursing/
Temporary Permit: Six months or until results of first exam are received and license is issued; $20
State Board Fee: $120
Additional State Endorsement: $120 plus $15 Criminal Release Authorization form
NCLEX-RN* Test Fee: $200

Re-Examination Limitations: Every 91 days
License Renewal: Birthday, every two years; $100
CEU Requirements: 30 contact hours every two years

New Jersey
Board of Nursing
P.O. Box 45010
Newark, NJ 07101
Phone: 973-504-6430
Fax: 973-648-3481
www.state.nj.us/oag/ca/medical/ nursing.htm
Temporary Permit: Not available
State Board Fee: $75 application fee plus $120 initial license fee
Additional State Endorsement: $75 application fee; $120 license certificate fee
NCLEX-RN° Test Fee: $200
Re-Examination Limitations: Every 91 days; only with remediation after three attempts
License Renewal: May 31, every two years; $120
CEU Requirements: None

New Mexico
Board of Nursing
6301 Indian School NE, Suite 710
Albuquerque, NM 87110
Phone: 505-841-8340
Fax: 505-841-8347
state.nm.us/clients/nursing
Temporary Permit: 24 weeks from graduation if application process is completed within 12 weeks of graduation; six months

if by endorsement. Fee is included in application fee; must have NM employment verified. If by endorsement, fee is $30.
State Board Fee: $110 initial exam
Additional State Endorsement: $110
NCLEX-RN° Test Fee: $200
Re-Examination Limitations: Every 91 days; $55
License Renewal: Every two years from date of issue; $93
CEU Requirements: 30 contact hours every two years

New York
Board of Nursing
NYS Education Department
Office of the Professions
Division of Professional Licensing Services, Nurse Unit
89 Washington Avenue
Albany, NY 12234-1000
Phone: 518-474-3817, ext. 280
Fax: 518-474-3398
op.nysed.gov/nurse.htm
Temporary Permit: Must have completed all other requirements for licensure except the licensing examination. Valid for one year from date of issue or until ten days after the applicant is notified of failure on the licensing examination, whichever occurs first. Graduates of New York state nursing programs may be employed without permit for 90 days immediately following graduation; $35
State Board Fee: $135 (includes first license and three-year registration)
Additional State Endorsement: $135

363

NCLEX-RN° Test Fee: $200
Re-Examination Limitations: Every 91 days
License Renewal: Every three years; $65
CEU Requirements: None

North Carolina
Board of Nursing
P.O. Box 2129
Raleigh, NC 27602-2129
Phone: 919-782-3211
Fax: 919-781-9461
ncbon.com
Temporary Permit: None for new graduates. By endorsement: six months or until the endorsement is approved, whichever occurs first; not renewable. Fee is included in application fee.
State Board Fee: $50
Additional State Endorsement: $150 plus $38 fingerprint fee
NCLEX-RN° Test Fee: $200
Re-Examination Limitations: Every 45 days; $40
License Renewal: Month of birth, every two years; $60
CEU Requirements: None

North Dakota
Board of Nursing
919 South 7th Street, Suite 504
Bismarck, ND 58504-5881
Phone: 701-328-9777
Fax: 701-328-9785
ndbon.org
Work Authorization: By endorsement: 90 days; fee is included in endorsement fee. By exam: 90 days after the date

of issue or upon notification of exam results, whichever occurs first.
You are not eligible for licensure in ND if your primary state of residence is AZ, AR, DE, ID, IA, ME, MD, MS, NM, NC, SD, TN, TX, UT, or WI. (Nurse Licensure Compact, 1/1/04)
State Board Fee: $110
Additional State Endorsement: $110
NCLEX-RN° Test Fee: $200
Re-Examination Limitations: Every 91 days, up to five attempts in three years
License Renewal: December 31, every even year; $90
CEU Requirements: Nursing practice for relicensure must meet or exceed 12 hours within preceding two years.

Ohio
Board of Nursing
17 South High Street, Suite 400
Columbus, OH 43215-7410
Phone: 614-466-3947
Fax: 614-466-0388
nursing.ohio.ogv
Temporary Permit: 180 days if by endorsement, not renewable. Fee is included in endorsement application fee.
State Board Fee: $75
Additional State Endorsement: $75
NCLEX-RN° Test Fee: $200
Re-Examination Limitations: Every 91 days; $75
License Renewal: August 31, every odd year; $65
CEU Requirements: 24 hours in a two-year period, except in the case of first renewal after licensure by examination.

Oklahoma

Board of Nursing
2915 North Classen Boulevard
Suite 524
Oklahoma City, OK 73106
Phone: 405-962-1800
Fax: 405-962-1821
youroklahoma.com/nursing/
Temporary Permit: 90 days if by
endorsement; $10
State Board Fee: $85
Additional State Endorsement: $85
NCLEX-RN° Test Fee: $200
Re-Examination Limitations: Every 91
days
License Renewal: Last day of birth
month, every even year; $75
CEU Requirements: None

Oregon

Board of Nursing
800 NE Oregon Street, Suite 465
Portland, OR 97232-2162
Phone: 971-673-0685
Fax: 971-673-0684
www.osbn.state.or.us/
Temporary Permit: None
State Board Fee: $100
Additional State Endorsement: $135
NCLEX-RN° Test Fee: $200
Re-Examination Limitations: Every 91
days, up to three years from the date of
graduation
License Renewal: Birthday, every two
years; $85
CEU Requirements: Nursing practice
for relicensure must exceed 960 hours
within preceding five years.

Pennsylvania

Board of Nursing
P.O. Box 2649
Harrisburg, PA 17105-2649
Phone: 717-783-7142
Fax: 717-783-0822
www.dos.state.pa.us/bpoa/site/default.asp
Temporary Permit: one year
maximum; examination results preempt
permit, $35
State Board Fee: $35 if educated in PA;
$100 if educated out of state
Additional State Endorsement: $100
NCLEX-RN° Test Fee: $200
Re-Examination Limitations: Every 91
days
License Renewal: Renewal date by
license number every two years; $45
CEU Requirements: None

Rhode Island

Board of Nurse Registration and
Nursing Education
3 Capitol Hill, Room 205
Providence, RI 02908
Phone: 401-222-5700
Fax: 401-222-3352
www.health.state.ri.us/hsr/professions/
nurses.php
Temporary Permit: Pending results
of first exam but no longer than 90
days after graduation; 90 days if by
endorsement. Not renewable. No fee.
State Board Fee: $93.75
Additional State Endorsement: $93.75
NCLEX-RN° Test Fee: $200
Re-Examination Limitations: Every 91
days

License Renewal: March 1, every two years by license number; $62.50
CEU Requirements: Beginning in March 2006, 10 contact hours in preceding two years.

South Carolina
Board of Nursing
P.O. Box 12367
Columbia, SC 29211-2367
Phone: 803-896-4550
Fax: 803-896-4525
www.llr.state.sc.us/pol/nursing/
Temporary Permit: 90 days by endorsement only; $10
State Board Fee: $97
Additional State Endorsement: $114; with permit $124
NCLEX-RN° Test Fee: $200
Re-Examination Limitations: Every 91 days, up to four times in one year, then must remediate; $65
License Renewal: April 30, every year; $64
CEU Requirements:
1. completion of thirty (30) contact hours from a continuing education provider recognized by the board; or
2. maintenance of certification or re-certification by a national certifying body recognized by the board; or
3. completion of an academic program of study in nursing or a related field recognized by the board; or
4. verification of competency and the number of hours practiced as evidenced by employer certification on a form approved by the Board.

South Dakota
Board of Nursing
4305 S. Louise Avenue, Suite 201
Sioux Falls, SD 57106-3115
Phone: 605-362-2760
Fax: 605-362-2768
www.state.sd.us/doh/nursing/
Temporary Permit: 90 days from graduation pending results of first exam; 90 days if by endorsement; $25
State Board Fee: $100
Additional State Endorsement: $100
NCLEX-RN° Test Fee: $200
Re-Examination Limitations: Every 91 days, maximum of four times per year in three years, then must requalify; $100
License Renewal: Birthday, every two years; $90
CEU Requirements: Continuing employment 140 hours in one year or 480 hours in six years.

Tennessee
Board of Nursing
425 Fifth Avenue North
Cordell Hull Building, 3rd Floor
Nashville, TN 37247-1010
Phone: 615-532-3202
Fax: 615-741-7899
www2.state.tn.us/health/Boards/Nursing/
Temporary Permit: Six months if by endorsement. Fee included in application fee.
State Board Fee: $140
Additional State Endorsement: $140
NCLEX-RN° Test Fee: $200

Re-Examination Limitations: Every 91 days, up to three years, then only with remediation
License Renewal: Last day of month of birth, every two years; $50
CEU Requirements: Continued practice requirement over a five-year period

Texas

Board of Nurse Examiners
333 Guadalupe #3-460
P.O. Box 430
Austin, TX 78701
Phone: 512-305-7400
Fax: 512-305-7401
bne.state.tx.us/
Temporary Permit: By endorsement: 12 weeks. By exam: 60 days or pending results of first exam. Fee included in application fee.
State Board Fee: $139
Additional State Endorsement: $200
NCLEX-RN® Test Fee: $200
Re-Examination Limitations: Every 45 days; unlimited testing within four years of eligibility; $70 retake fee
License Renewal: Every even year for those born in even years, every odd year for those born in odd years (initial licensure period ranges from six months to 29 months depending on birth year); $67
CEU Requirements: 20 contact hours (2 CEUs) every two years. Nurses licensed by exam or by endorsement are exempt from CE requirements for the first renewal after initial licensure.

Utah

Board of Nursing
Division of Occupational and Professional Licensing
P.O. Box 146741
Salt Lake City, UT 84114-6741
Phone: 801-530-6628
Fax: 801-530-6511
commerce.utah.gov/opl/licensing/nurse.html
Temporary Permit: Four months; $50
State Board Fee: $99
Additional State Endorsement: $99
NCLEX-RN® Test Fee: $200
Re-Examination Limitations: Every 45 days; those who fail to pass exam within two years after completing educational program must submit plan of action for approval before retaking
License Renewal: January 31, every odd year; $58
CEU Requirements: Must have practiced not less than 400 hours during two years preceding application for renewal, or have completed 30 contact hours, or have practiced not less than 200 hours and completed 15 contact hours during two years preceding application for renewal.

Vermont

Board of Nursing
Office of the Secretary of State
81 River Street
Montpelier, VT 05609-1106
Phone: 802-828-2396
Fax: 802-828-2484
vtprofessionals.org/OPR1/nurses/
Temporary Permit: 90 days if by endorsement; $25

State Board Fee: $90
Additional State Endorsement: $150
NCLEX-RN® Test Fee: $200
Re-Examination Limitations: Every 91 days; Board of Nursing approval is needed after two attempts; $30
License Renewal: March 31, every odd year; $85
CEU Requirements: Minimum practice requirement of 960 hours in five years or 400 hours in two years

Virginia

Board of Nursing
6603 West Broad Street, 5th Floor
Richmond, VA 23230-1712
Phone: 804-662-9909
Fax: 804-662-9512
www.dhp.state.va.us/nursing/
Temporary Permit: 90 days pending results of exam
State Board Fee: $130
Additional State Endorsement: $130
NCLEX-RN® Test Fee: $200
Re-Examination Limitations: Every 91 days; $25
License Renewal: Last day of month of birth, every even year for those born in even years, every odd year for those born in odd years; $95
CEU Requirements: None

Washington

Nursing Care Quality Assurance Commission
310 Israel Road
Tumwater, WA 98501-7860

Mailing Address (for payments)
Health Professions Quality Assurance
Customer Service Center
P.O. Box 1099
Olympia, WA 98507-1099
Mailing Address (not for payments)
Health Professions Quality Assurance
Customer Service Center
P.O. Box 47865
Olympia, WA 98504
Phone: 360-236-4700
Fax: 360-236-4818
www.doh.wa.gov/licensing.htm#N
Temporary Permit: None
State Board Fee: $70
Additional State Endorsement: $70
NCLEX-RN® Test Fee: $200
Re-Examination Limitations: Every 91 days, up to three times in two years, then must requalify
License Renewal: Birthday, every year; Normally $55; reduced to $50 from July 1, 2006 to June 30, 2007
CEU Requirements: Not mandatory

West Virginia

Board of Examiners for Registered Professional Nurses
101 Dee Drive, Suite 102
Charleston, WV 25311-1620
Phone: 304-558-3596
Fax: 304-558-3666
wvrnboard.com
Temporary Permit: 90 days pending results of first exam; 90 days if by endorsement; $10
State Board Fee: $51.50
Additional State Endorsement: $60
NCLEX-RN® Test Fee: $200

Re-Examination Limitations: Every 91 days; additional requirements are needed after two attempts
License Renewal: December 31, every year; $25
CEU Requirements: 30 contact hours every odd year. If initial licensure occurs during the first half of any two-year reporting period: must complete 12 contact hours before the end of that reporting period. If initial licensure occurs during the second half of any two-year reporting period: exempt from CE requirements for the entire reporting period.

Wisconsin

Bureau of Health Service Professions—RN
Department of Regulation and Licensing
1400 East Washington Avenue
P.O. Box 8935
Madison, WI 53708-8935
Phone: 608-266-2112
Fax: 608-261-7083
drl.wi.gov/prof/rn/def.htm
Temporary Permit: Three months pending results of exam; three months if by endorsement; $10
State Board Fee: $68
Additional State Endorsement: $66
NCLEX-RN® Test Fee: $200
Re-Examination Limitations: Every 45 days; $15
License Renewal: February 28 or 29, every even year; $66
CEU Requirements: None

Wyoming

Board of Nursing
1810 Pioneer Avenue
Cheyenne, WY 82002
Phone: 307-777-7601
Fax: 307-777-3519
nursing.state.wy.us/
Temporary Permit: 90 days by endorsement or by exam. Fee is included in application fee.
State Board Fee: $190
Additional State Endorsement: $195
NCLEX-RN® Test Fee: $200
Re-Examination Limitations: Every 91 days, maximum of 10 times within five years of graduation
License Renewal: December 31, every even year; $110
CEU Requirements: Minimum practice requirement of 1,600 hours in five years or 500 hours in two years.

A SPECIAL NOTE FOR INTERNATIONAL NURSES

If you are not from the United States but are interested in learning more about American nursing, wish to practice in the United States, or are exploring the possibilities of attending an American nursing school for graduate study, Kaplan can help you.

To function as a registered nurse in the United States, it is necessary for you to become licensed as a R.N. by a state board of nursing. Many U.S. state boards of nursing require internationally educated nurses to obtain a certificate from the Commission on Graduates of Foreign Nursing Schools (CGFNS®) before applying for initial licensure as a registered nurse. The process of obtaining a CGFNS® certificate includes (1) review of your nursing credentials and original nursing education program, (2) passing the CGFNS® exam that tests nursing knowledge, and (3) obtaining a minimum score on an English-language proficiency examination.

Kaplan offers comprehensive courses of study to help you pass the CGFNS® and English-language proficiency exams. To obtain course information please call 1-800-533-8850. Outside the U.S.A. please call 1-213-452-5700 or log onto the website at *kaplannursing.com*.

Applications for the CGFNS® exam are free and can be obtained by calling CGFNS® at 215-349-8767. To find out about a particular state's requirements for international nurses, call that state's board of nursing and request an application packet for initial licensure as an internationally educated nurse. The websites for each of the State Boards of Nursing in the United States are listed in the previous resource.

Once you have a CGFNS® certificate, it is necessary for you to take and pass the NCLEX-RN® exam (National Council Licensure Examination). You should apply to the state board of nursing in the state in which you wish to practice nursing to take the NCLEX-RN® exam.

Kaplan has comprehensive course and review products to help you pass the NCLEX-RN® exam. To obtain course information please call 1-800-533-8850. Outside the United States, please call 1-213-452-5700 or log onto the website at *kaplannursing.com*.

Additional Resources for International Students and Professionals

In addition to courses to prepare for the registered nurse licensure exams, Kaplan provides international students and professionals programs to develop the English language skills necessary to study or work in the United States. Course offerings include intensive English, Pre-MBA studies, and standardized exam preparation for such exams as the SAT®, TOEFL®, GMAT®, and GRE®. With campus and city centers across the U.S.A., Kaplan has a location perfect for everyone. Call 1-800-527-8378. Or, outside the U.S.A., call 1-213-452-5800.

Kaplan is authorized under U.S. federal law to enroll nonimmigrant alien students.

Test names are registered trademarks of their respective owners.

Notes

Notes